Coping with Bronchitis and Emphysema

Dr Tom Smith has been writing since 1977, after spending six years in general practice and seven years in medical research. He writes the 'Doctor, Doctor' column in the *Guardian* on Saturdays, and has written three humorous books, *Doctor, Have You Got a Minute?*, *A Seaside Practice* and *Going Loco*, all published by Short Books. His other books for Sheldon Press include *Heart Attacks: Prevent and Survive*, *Living with Alzheimer's Disease*, *Overcoming Back Pain*, *Coping with Bowel Cancer*, *Coping with Heartburn and Reflux*, *Coping with Age-related Memory Loss*, *Skin Cancer: Prevent and Survive*, *How to Get the Best from Your Doctor*, *Coping with Kidney Disease*, *Osteoporosis: Prevent and Treat* and *Coping Successfully with Prostate Cancer*.

Overcoming Common Problems Series

Selected titles

A full list of titles is available from Sheldon Press,
36 Causton Street, London SW1P 4ST and on our website at
www.sheldonpress.co.uk

Asperger Syndrome in Adults
Dr Ruth Searle

The Assertiveness Handbook
Mary Hartley

Assertiveness: Step by step
Dr Windy Dryden and Daniel Constantinou

Backache: What you need to know
Dr David Delvin

Body Language: What you need to know
David Cohen

Bulimia, Binge-eating and their Treatment
Professor J. Hubert Lacey, Dr Bryony Bamford and
Amy Brown

The Cancer Survivor's Handbook
Dr Terry Priestman

The Chronic Pain Diet Book
Neville Shone

Cider Vinegar
Margaret Hills

Confidence Works
Gladeana McMahon

Coping Successfully with Pain
Neville Shone

Coping Successfully with Prostate Cancer
Dr Tom Smith

Coping Successfully with Psoriasis
Christine Craggs-Hinton

Coping Successfully with Ulcerative Colitis
Peter Cartwright

Coping Successfully with Varicose Veins
Christine Craggs-Hinton

Coping Successfully with Your Hiatus Hernia
Dr Tom Smith

Coping Successfully with Your Irritable Bowel
Rosemary Nicol

Coping When Your Child Has Cerebral Palsy
Jill Eckersley

Coping with Age-related Memory Loss
Dr Tom Smith

**Coping with Birth Trauma and Postnatal
Depression**
Lucy Jolin

Coping with Bowel Cancer
Dr Tom Smith

Coping with Candida
Shirley Trickett

Coping with Chemotherapy
Dr Terry Priestman

Coping with Chronic Fatigue
Trudie Chalder

Coping with Coeliac Disease
Karen Brody

Coping with Compulsive Eating
Dr Ruth Searle

**Coping with Diabetes in Childhood and
Adolescence**
Dr Philippa Kaye

Coping with Diverticulitis
Peter Cartwright

Coping with Dyspraxia
Jill Eckersley

Coping with Early-onset Dementia
Jill Eckersley

Coping with Eating Disorders and Body Image
Christine Craggs-Hinton

Coping with Envy
Dr Windy Dryden

**Coping with Epilepsy in Children and Young
People**
Susan Elliot-Wright

Coping with Family Stress
Dr Peter Cheevers

Coping with Gout
Christine Craggs-Hinton

Coping with Hay Fever
Christine Craggs-Hinton

Coping with Headaches and Migraine
Alison Frith

Coping with Hearing Loss
Christine Craggs-Hinton

Coping with Heartburn and Reflux
Dr Tom Smith

Coping with Kidney Disease
Dr Tom Smith

Overcoming Common Problems Series

Overcoming Common Problems Series

Overcoming Common Problems

Coping with Bronchitis and Emphysema

Second edition

DR TOM SMITH

sheldon **PRESS**

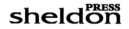

First published in Great Britain in 1994

Sheldon Press
36 Causton Street
London SW1P 4ST
www.sheldonpress.co.uk

Reprinted three times
Second edition published 2011

Illustrations by Alasdair Smith

British Library Cataloguing-in-Publication Data
A catalogue record for this book is available from the British Library

ISBN 978-1-84709-152-9

1 3 5 7 9 10 8 6 4 2

Typeset by Fakenham Photosetting Ltd, Fakenham, Norfolk
Printed in Great Britain by Ashford Colour Press

Produced on paper from sustainable forests

Contents

Acknowledgements and note to the reader

Acknowledgements

I would like to thank the following:

Lesley Munro, of Chest Heart and Stroke Scotland, who encouraged me and gave me much useful information;

Julia Smith, of the British Lung Foundation, for her kind interest and enthusiasm;

Dr George Hearn, my old 'boss', who, as Consultant Chest Physician at Dudley Road Hospital, Birmingham, led his housemen by example – his care for his patients has been my model for more than thirty years;

The doctors and staff at Stranraer Health Centre, Scotland, for I could not have had better or more supportive colleagues and friends.

Note to the reader

This is not a medical book and is not intended to replace advice from your doctor. Consult your pharmacist or doctor if you believe you have any of the symptoms described, and if you think you might need medical help.

Introduction: a view from 2010

When the first edition of this book was planned in the 1990s, my publishers and I discussed the title in detail. Then, chronic lung disease was still generally known as chronic bronchitis and emphysema. So we decided to use that term in our title – *Coping with Bronchitis and Emphysema*, although through the book we also used the term chronic obstructive airways disease (also known by the acronym COAD). Now, in 2010, the public know this condition as chronic obstructive pulmonary disease (COPD). So, while the book retains the same title, we now tend to use COPD when discussing this disease. However, the book's main message remains the same, and much of it, happily, does not need to be rewritten. What has changed is the evidence base on which general practitioners like myself have decided to manage our patients with COPD, and how you, the patients, and your carers respond to us.

There is now a massive literature on which we can build our treatments for COPD, in particular on how we can help to prevent the repeated lung infections that are the bane of your lives, and which slowly and inexorably continue to damage your lungs. The final chapter of this book reviews this latest evidence, so that you can understand fully why your doctors manage your illness in the way they do.

One message above all has been proven beyond all doubt. In the first decade of this new century, first Ireland, then Scotland and finally the rest of the United Kingdom, banned smoking in public. Within a year of the ban in each country in turn the numbers of deaths from heart and lung disease dropped significantly, saving thousands of lives. The benefit was highest in those who were passive smokers – such as non-smoking bartenders and the spouses of smokers. If ever the terrible damage inflicted by smoking were in doubt, no one can harbour that doubt today. Doctors can help you hugely with your lung disease, with modern treatments, medical and physical, but all is to no avail if you continue to smoke. What I wrote in the 1990s is still relevant today.

Just as significant a change since the 1990s is the way medical practices all over the country have organized themselves to follow up and monitor illnesses. General practitioners have taken it upon themselves to provide lung and heart clinics, run from their health centres and manned by specialist nurses and the doctors themselves. We are watching much more closely than ever before the progress of people with COPD, and fine-tuning their treatments to deal with their changing circumstances. This gradual switch from hospital to general practice care is bound to continue, as family doctors take more responsibility for specialist care. Part of the change is economic: it is far cheaper to the National Health Service for GPs to look after patients than for hospital clinicians to do so. But partly it is because it is much easier for the patients to be looked after locally, and more satisfying for their family doctors to take on the responsibility, provided we have the tools and knowledge to do it well.

In 2010, caring for people with COPD is now the job of the community health team. This team encompasses the skills of doctors, nurses, physiotherapists and occupational health professionals. We work together to get the optimum results for our patients, and most of the time we succeed. This book explains how we try to do so. If you are worried about your future with COPD, I do hope it helps.

Introduction to the first edition

This book is for everyone who coughs regularly. You may think it is normal or natural to cough, say, first thing in the morning or when you have broken into a short run or had to walk faster than usual, but it isn't. You may think it is normal to cough through the winter, and to improve in the spring and summer, but it isn't. You may think that a cough to 'clear the tubes' after a cigarette is natural, but it isn't.

Having a cough regularly – one that persists even when you do not have a cold or 'catarrh' – is a sign of something going wrong inside your chest. Usually that something is chronic bronchitis, often it can be emphysema, and sometimes it can be asthma. Rarely, today, it may be tuberculosis, and, very occasionally, it can be an early sign of something much worse, like lung cancer.

So, a chronic cough should not be taken lightly. If you are bothered by a cough, even if it is only for a few weeks in the year or a few minutes every morning, then you need to do something about it. Doctors can only do so much in terms of treatment and advice. The effort must be made by you, even if it means a complete change of lifestyle and abandoning lifelong habits. Take the plunge now and the improvement that you make in your health should last you into a fit and active old age. Let the chance pass by, however, and from your mid forties onwards, your 'bad chest' will make you increasingly chair-bound.

The same goes for the other 'chesty' problem that goes hand in hand with the cough – breathlessness.

Do you quickly run out of puff when you break into a run, say, when you have to cross the street in a hurry? Are you a bit breathless when you walk up a slight slope or even on the level? When you walk upstairs, do you have to rest on the landing or hold on to the banisters for a while half-way up?

A fit 50 year old can run 6 miles in an hour on the flat at a steady pace without being too puffed. Could you hope to approach this speed for even half this time or do you forget the last time you ever broke into more than a gentle stroll?

If these problems strike a chord, then this book is for you. It explains how you breathe, how the lungs work, what can go wrong with them, and why. It concentrates on the two commonest chesty conditions: bronchitis and emphysema. Doctors now refer to them jointly as COPD, but, as this term overlaps with conditions such as asthma, cystic fibrosis and work-related chest disease, and the way we try to ease them all is the same, these other problems are given some space here, too.

The main message is that something can always be done for a 'bad chest', provided we obey the rules. The best way of obeying the rules is to understand why they have been set. So, although the medical treatments for COPD are presented in full, it is vital – if you are going to give your lungs any chance to improve – to follow the guidance in the chapters on smoking and exercise. We can fight damaged airways, and help the lungs to repair themselves, with cleaner air, medicines, and physiotherapy and even, at times, with surgery, but there is no chance of success if they are constantly filled with smoke and you remain a couch potato!

So, read on and help your doctor to help you to a healthier future.

1

Breathing

We take a breath around 12 times a minute every minute of our lives, yet we are hardly ever aware of it. Now you have had the act of breathing brought to your attention, though, think about it for a while.

How do we breathe?

You know you are sucking in air through your nose (if you are using your mouth, then you already have a problem), but what muscles are you using to do so?

If you are reading this while sitting and relaxed, then all the 'suck' force you need is supplied by a gentle expansion of your ribcage, say a couple of centimetres or so. As the chest expands, this opens up the airways inside and, as nature abhors a vacuum, air rushes in through the nose, through the airways in the back of the throat and chest, to reach the delicate 'sacs' in the depths of the lungs, where they expand like tiny balloons.

You breathe out simply by allowing the expanded ribcage muscles to relax. This reduces the volume inside the chest, so that the balloon-like sacs empty of air, which then flows out again through the airways and nose.

This is nice and simple so far, but what happens when you need more air? The first step is to expand your chest even more, simply by using those ribcage muscles, because the more you open them up, the more air will rush into your chest. You also utilize the diaphragm, the tough sheet of muscle that divides the chest from the abdomen. (You are probably only conscious of moving your diaphragm when you hiccup, which is a sudden spasm or cramp of the diaphragm.) Contract your diaphragm and it moves downwards, expanding the space in which the lungs lie downwards as well as outwards, thus inhaling more air.

What if you need more air still? Then, your nose is no longer wide enough to take in all the air you need above, so you begin to gulp it in through your mouth. Also the ribs and diaphragm may not be giving you enough space inside your chest, so you use the big muscles that run from the neck to the shoulders and the top of the breastbone – the ones that enable you to turn your head and shrug – to help open the chest further. This makes your shoulders rise and the big neck muscles on either side of your throat bulge with each breath. You may have to hold on to something, to give these muscles more leverage, so that you can expand your chest to its maximum. Look at athletes after an exhausting race, and you will see them holding on to a post, so that they can 'get their breath back'.

This is the normal sequence of events when we exert ourselves. Take as an example a brisk run. We start by breathing normally, but, as we begin to use up the energy in our muscles, they demand more oxygen. We breathe faster and more deeply until we are using all the muscles we have to keep the oxygen supply going. At some point in the run we become acutely aware that we are breathless and this can even make us feel distressed. However, if we are fit and well trained, we can 'run through' this phase, into the 'second wind'. The less fit we are, the sooner we hit this distressed phase, the longer it lasts, and the longer we take to recover from it – and the less likely we are to achieve that comforting second wind.

To be frank, we do not actually know what this second wind is; indeed, some doctors even argue that it does not exist. It may simply be the result of the conscious part of the brain deciding to ignore the signals of distress it is receiving from the lungs, so that breathing returns to being a mechanism that is more automatic than conscious. Whatever causes it, athletes experience it either during a run or in the warm-up beforehand, and they know that it is a sign of fitness.

The point is that fitness and training are vital for athletes, to keep their lungs in trim and to improve their performance. These factors are even more important for people with long-term lung diseases, such as bronchitis and emphysema. The more they use their lungs, the healthier they will be.

Many people with chronic coughs or those who easily become breathless will recognize themselves in this description of what happens when people run – except that it occurs when they are at rest or when they are walking about doing the routine things of everyday life. In fact, they may be in a constant state of second wind, in that, even at rest, they are breathing harder and faster than normal, but do not notice it. The brain is no longer heeding the warning signals from their overworked lungs. Their relatives and friends notice, however. People with COPD can be remarkably breathless and seem to be in real distress, yet they may not *feel* breathless until someone brings it to their attention. Often it is only then that they become concerned themselves.

We all know we have to keep breathing to survive (if we stop breathing for as little as four minutes we die). Understanding *why* this should be so is essential for anyone wishing to care for their lungs.

Why do we need to breathe?

Oxygen is essential to every cell and tissue in our bodies: it is our fuel; we use it in all the processes that keep us active and conscious. If we are deprived of oxygen, our hearts stop within a few seconds, we become unconscious in a minute or two, and the brain is permanently damaged only a few minutes later. Death follows soon afterwards.

Breathing is our only way of obtaining oxygen. To keep up the correct levels of oxygen in our bodies, before we even start to do anything, we must process about 0.5 litre (1 pint) of air through our lungs about 12 times a minute, every minute of the day and night. With exertion, the requirement rises to about 1.5 litres ($2^1/_2$ pints) 30 times a minute. About a fifth of the air we breathe is oxygen, and our lungs are specifically designed to 'capture' it from the air and pass it very rapidly into the bloodstream.

On its way towards the lungs, however, the air is ingeniously processed, so that nothing but air, at body temperature, with the correct moisture content, and without dusts, pollens, irritants or germs, reaches the vital areas where the transfer of oxygen to the circulation takes place.

What happens when we breathe?

The nose and throat

The nose is the first step. When we breathe in, the air is wafted over the 'turbinate' bones (see Figure 1), which are ledges that protrude into the air spaces inside the nostrils. They do exactly what their name suggests: they cause eddies in the air current so that all the air entering the nose must come into direct contact with their surfaces. If there is anything solid in that air, such as particles of dust or pollen, it will stick to these surfaces. So, the nose's first function is to filter the air, preventing pollutants from passing lower down into the chest.

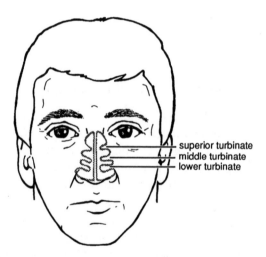

superior turbinate
middle turbinate
lower turbinate

Figure 1 The nose – filter, warmer, moisturizer

It has two other vital purposes: it brings the entering air to the correct body temperature, so that no matter the temperature of the outside air – be it freezing cold or tropical – it enters the lungs at just the right level of warmth. It also corrects the moisture content of the air. Breathe in dry air and your nose will do its best to add moisture to it, to keep the lungs comfortable.

So, when you are breathing normally, your nose tries to make sure that the air entering your lungs is pure, warm, and moist, to give the best possible conditions for oxygen to be transferred into your bloodstream.

This is why breathing in through your mouth is less healthy. Your mouth has no filtering turbinates or specialized warming and moisturizing chambers, and what you breathe in through it goes straight into the lungs, unprepared. Chronic mouth breathers need advice on how to restore their noses to their proper function.

It is also why smoking does so much damage. Smokers do not stick their cigarettes up their noses, for the very good reason that the hot smoke, direct from a cigarette, would irritate the sensitive membranes inside the nostrils and on the turbinate bones beyond belief. The surfaces inside the nose are sensitive to irritants, unlike the inside lining of the airways in the chest, which are devoid of nerves that can transmit the sensation of pain.

Worse still, smokers, by bypassing the nose, deliver air to the chest that is low in oxygen (it is used up in burning the tobacco), devoid of moisture (it, too, is burned away), but high in ash, tars and irritant solids, some particles of which are still glowing at around 400°C (752°F)! If this were not enough, highly poisonous carbon monoxide and nicotine accompany them.

When you inhale cigarette smoke, this disastrous combination first hits the tongue, then, in order, the back of the throat, the larynx (voice-box) and the main air passages from the larynx into the chest – the trachea and bronchi. All these structures have very delicate surfaces, not designed to cope with such concentrated pollution, and they react in the best way they can.

Often, sadly, their best is not good enough, and it is easy to understand why. Neither the trachea, the main 'windpipe' in the throat, nor the bronchi, the main airways in the chest, are primarily designed to filter and regulate the content of the air entering the lungs because this is the nose's job. The trachea and bronchi are there to conduct the air into the deeper reaches of the lungs, where the vital oxygen exchange takes place.

The trachea and bronchi

All the upper air passages – the nose, throat and larynx – are highly sensitive to irritation and inflammation, which is why the throat is so sore and it hurts when you swallow when you have tonsillitis. It also explains the tickliness and discomfort you feel when you have a cold, when the nose and throat are inflamed. When you have hay fever, you are congested and have a fiery, tickling sensation in the eyes, nose, and throat because all these areas are super-sensitive to pollen. Laryngitis can be the most uncomfortable of all, making you sore, tickly and hoarse, all at the same time.

Less common is tracheitis (inflammation of the trachea), which can give you a sore windpipe, deep in the throat, but the trachea is, as a rule, much less sensitive than the nose and throat.

Any inflammation below the trachea, from the bronchi down, can be quite 'silent', by which is meant that you do not feel it at all. This is because the bronchi and lungs themselves do not contain any nerves of sensation, so disease can grumble along inside them and you are completely unaware of it. Maybe this is why so many smokers do not really believe that smoking is bad for them. Because they do not feel any bad effects immediately, they assume that nothing is happening, that they are perfectly healthy. Nothing could be further from the truth. For some people who have fairly advanced chronic bronchitis, whose bronchi have been inflamed for many years, the only symptom may be a morning cough, which they immediately assume to be a normal part of life.

The trachea is the large gristly tube you can feel in the centre of your throat below your Adam's apple (the larynx). It is kept open by horseshoe-shaped bands of cartilage, interspersed with muscle and elastic-type tissue, so it can expand and contract with each breath.

Deep in the chest, the trachea divides into the two main bronchi, one to each lung. The bigger bronchi contain in their walls muscle, elastic tissue and cartilage, like the trachea, and are narrower. They, in turn, divide into smaller and smaller bronchi as they reach deeper into their respective lungs, resembling the branches of a tree (see Figure 2). Each lung has ten main bronchial segments, each of which branches yet again into from 15 to 25 smaller bronchi.

The cartilage in the walls of the bigger bronchi acts as a supporting 'skeleton', keeping them open. The smaller bronchi, with

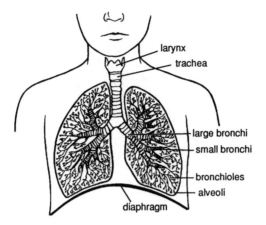

Figure 2 The bronchial tree

less cartilage in them, can collapse. Beyond the smaller bronchi are the bronchioles, which are like the 'twigs' off the bronchial 'tree'. Their walls are very thin and contain no cartilage, so they can collapse easily.

It is crucial to an understanding of chest diseases like COPD and emphysema to realize that in normal breathing, air flows freely all the way from the trachea to the bronchioles (see Figure 3 overleaf). The transfer of oxygen from the lungs to the bloodstream happens only in the smallest airways, the alveoli or air sacs, beyond the bronchioles. Bronchitis affects the bronchi, down to the bronchioles, while emphysema affects the alveoli, but more about this in the next chapter.

Apart from being the channel for air, the bronchial tree has another vital function. It is the lungs' last line of defence against particles of dust and pollen, and germs, in the air we breathe.

Knowing how it mounts this defence is the key to understanding bronchitis, which, put simply, is the result of the breakdown of the bronchial defence mechanism.

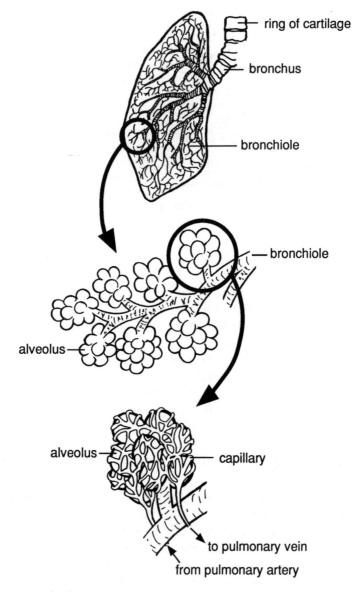

Figure 3 The lungs

Defending the lungs

The inner surfaces of the bronchi are lined with two types of cells: 'hairy' (the medical term is ciliated) cells and 'goblet' cells (see Figure 4). The hairs of the ciliated cells protrude into the airway and their purpose is to catch any foreign material that has passed by the nose and, by 'wafting' it upwards, to transport it up and out of the lungs. The ciliated cells work in unison, so that waves of co-ordinated cilia pass from the depths of the lungs towards the larynx. Ingenious cine-microscopy of the inside of bronchi shows that the cilia of many thousands of cells move in much the same way as a field of wheat in the wind.

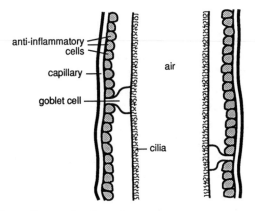

Figure 4 A bronchus under the microscope

Under the microscope, goblet cells look just like the wine glasses after which they are named, with their 'rims' towards the open airway. In a normal lung, they are few and far between – the ciliated cells dominate. Goblet cells secrete mucus into the airway, so that the bronchi have a very thin covering of fluid. This helps to trap unwanted particles from the air, and eases their passage out of the lung. The mucus flows upwards on the cilia to reach the larynx, where it is normally swallowed, quite unconsciously.

There is a third line of bronchial defence. Just under the surface of the bronchi is a network of blood vessels lying in a bed of tissue that is stuffed with a variety of 'inflammatory' cells, the sole purpose of which is to protect the body from invasion by bacteria, viruses and other foreign material, such as chemical irritants, that might be in the air. Many of these cells have counterparts in the white blood cells that protect the rest of the body against infection, but the fact that they are crammed into the tissues around the bronchi emphasizes how important the lungs' defence systems are. They would not be there in such concentration if they were not needed.

If the first two defences – the cilia and the mucus – have been breached, say by an infecting germ, then this third line comes into play. If they have been damaged, say by smoking (a single inhalation of cigarette smoke kills off many thousands of cilia), then the potential for severe harm to the integrity of the lung is immense. What happens to these defence systems in bronchitis will be explained in the next chapter. Suffice to say meanwhile that in cases of chronic bronchitis, there are many fewer ciliated cells, and many more goblet cells, so there is much more mucus to bring up, and the mechanism to transport it out of the lungs is much less efficient. This explains, in part, why the person with bronchitis needs to cough – if the cilia are not working, then you have to cough to remove the excess mucus.

Thus, regularly coughing in the morning is a first sign that your lungs' defences are weakening – your population of cilia are disappearing, and your goblet cells are overworking and multiplying. Your inflammatory cells are being irritated and stimulating you to cough. If you do not 'explode' the excess mucus out of your lungs, your smaller airways will be blocked with fluid. They may collapse down, under the suction pressure of the mucus inside them. To get air to pass beyond them, you must cough to clear them. If you cannot clear them, air will not reach the alveoli and you will not be able to use that part of the lung to oxygenate the blood.

The message, then, is clear: if you have a chronic cough, then your first lines of defence are already under threat and you must take action. What this action should be is described in later chapters.

The alveoli

The final destination of the air we breathe in is the alveoli. These are air sacs (they look like tiny bubbles) separated from each other only by the thinnest of tissue, through which many small blood vessels – called capillaries – wind. In the act of breathing, these 'bubbles' expand and contract. Oxygen passes from the air into the capillaries and carbon dioxide, formed in our bodies as a waste product of every living activity, passes in the other direction, to be expelled in our exhaled breath.

The alveoli open at birth, with our first breath, and are kept open because they contain a fluid called surfactant – a form of natural detergent that, because it has a very low surface tension, prevents the opposite walls of the alveoli from sticking together. Thus, premature babies, born before the surfactant has time to form, have great difficulty in breathing because their alveoli cannot open up properly. In recent years, they have been given artificial surfactant (in the form of drops or a spray into the lungs), a treatment that has saved many thousands of babies' lives. Some types of emphysema in adults may be due to lack of, or abnormal, surfactant, a possibility that may lead to treatments for the disease being developed in the future.

The main structures of the lungs are complete by the time we are born, but new alveoli continue to form for another eight years afterwards, their numbers increasing from 20 million at birth to 300 million. From then on, no new alveoli form, but the existing ones increase in diameter and, more particularly, in surface area as the ribcage develops.

The surface area of our alveoli (see Figure 5 overleaf) is very important, as it is the only surface through which we can take in oxygen. So, the larger the surface area, and the more efficient it is, the better is our ability to take in oxygen from the air. A normal adult alveolus measures, on average, 0.25 millimetre across. Spread out, the total surface area of all the alveoli in one person's lungs would cover a square 75 by 75 metres (82 yards) or, roughly, the surface area of a football pitch. All the protective mechanisms in the nose, throat, and bronchi, described above, are designed to drive the maximum amount of oxygen at the best possible temperature

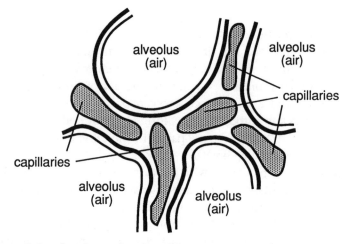

Figure 5 An alveolus under the microscope

and moisture, with the least possible pollution on to this 'football pitch' of alveolar surface.

When we are healthy, this system is remarkably efficient. What happens, though, when the system goes wrong, as it does in cases of bronchitis and emphysema, for example, and what can we do to minimize and reverse the damage? Chapters 2 and 3 will answer these questions.

2

When breathing goes wrong: bronchitis, emphysema, bronchiectasis and related diseases

Introduction

The description 'chronic bronchitis and emphysema' has been used for years in the UK for smokers or ex-smokers who cough, bring up copious amounts of phlegm with the cough, and are breathless after relatively minor exertion, the type of exertion that would not bother the average person. This has largely been replaced by the term COPD, mainly because it was always difficult to separate the relative parts played by its two components – bronchitis and emphysema – in any particular individual.

Chronic bronchitis

'Chronic' simply means a process that is continuing, and does so steadily for a long time – for months and years rather than days. 'Bronchitis' means inflammation, infection or irritation of the bronchi. Chronic bronchitis, therefore, is responsible for the excess of mucus seen in most patients with bronchitis and emphysema. The bronchial walls are thickened by masses of inflammatory cells, many of the ciliated cells are destroyed, and there are many more mucus-producing goblet cells. The result is considerable narrowing of the larger bronchi, and the airway in some of the smaller bronchi can be completely blocked by a combination of the thickened walls and the excess of fluid inside the airway. Obviously less air can reach the alveoli beyond the narrowed or blocked bronchi.

Emphysema

In emphysema, the damage is to the alveoli. The alveoli have lots of tiny 'bubbles' (see Figure 6a), but in emphysema many of the tiny 'bubbles' are burst, so that the walls between them no longer exist (see Figure 6b). This means that there is less surface area for oxygen exchange between the air and the circulation, and fewer normal capillaries to take up this oxygen. The brain responds to the lack of oxygen by making you breathe harder and faster, and you become breathless.

Bronchiectasis

Some mention must be made here of this disease. In this common form of COPD, one or two branches of the bronchial tree are *widened* rather than narrowed and the affected bronchi produce much more mucus than normal. The mucus collects in the lung beyond the affected site, blocking the entry of air, and making this segment of lung more prone to infection.

In most adults who have bronchiectasis, it is confined to the lowest regions of the lung and there is no obvious cause. Other cases develop after an infection, which perhaps occurred years before, that has weakened the lung or caused explosive coughing. Tuberculosis used to be a common cause of bronchiectasis; now it is more likely to follow childhood measles or whooping cough (pertussis). Indeed, the prevention of bronchiectasis is a very good reason for vaccinating against whooping cough. Less commonly, bronchiectasis can follow influenza or pneumonia.

Bronchiectasis is a very common complication of cystic fibrosis. It is also the main problem in a rare inherited disorder called Kartagener's syndrome, in which all the organs are on the opposite side to normal, that is, the heart is on the right, the liver on the left, the appendix on the left, and so on. For those with this syndrome, the cilia on the bronchi do not appear to work normally. Strangely, Kartagener's syndrome may affect several family members in the same generation, such as brothers, sisters, and cousins, but has not

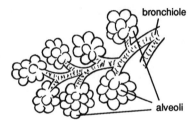

Figure 6a Healthy alveoli

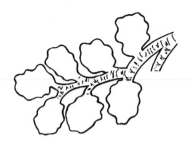

Figure 6b Alveoli in emphysema

been seen in more than one generation in the same family (children, nephews and nieces).

People with bronchiectasis cough a lot, and produce a lot of sputum (as much as a cupful every morning). The sputum sometimes contains rusty streaks of blood. Other symptoms include breathlessness, weight loss and weakness.

Of course, if your doctor has said that you have chronic bronchitis and emphysema or COPD or bronchiectasis, this all sounds frightening. You will be wondering 'Why me?, and is there a cure?' or, more positively, 'What can I do to help myself?' Happily, you can do a lot, and so can your doctor, if necessary. The rest of this book is about how to keep COPD at bay, and it is optimistic. But, before this, your first question – 'Why me?' – needs answering.

The causes of bronchitis, emphysema and COPD

Smoking

Far and away the most important cause of COPD is tobacco smoking. A few cases are caused by air pollution and constant exposure to bronchial irritants at work, and a very small proportion of cases (just under one in every hundred) is inherited. Some cases of COPD in adults may be the result of childhood chest infections caused by a particular germ, Haemophilus influenzae type B (HIB), which is why it is important to immunize children against it, but the fact remains, and cannot be emphasized too strongly, that smoking is the primary lung destroyer and has no peer.

By the time they are 11 years old, 10 per cent of British school-children who admit to smoking already have 'simple chronic bronchitis', which is defined as consisting of a persistent cough and phlegm due to the changes described above in the larger bronchi that occur as a result of smoking. These children, like older people with this form of bronchitis, are already prone to repeated chest infections. At this stage, however, if they stop smoking, the cough will disappear and they will come to no long-term harm. They do not yet have emphysema.

How smoking hurts the lung – the Dutch versus the British

The researchers are divided into two camps – the Dutch and the British views – about how smoking and other irritants cause COPD. The Dutch believe that its sufferers have an 'asthmatic predisposi-tion' that makes them react to smoke and other pollutants in the air with an allergic response in the bronchi, similar to that of asthma, but not as readily reversible. They point to the fact that adults who have had asthma as children are unusually susceptible to COPD in later life. They propose that the disease is at one extreme of the asthmatic process, in which cigarette smoke provokes an inflamma-tion of the lungs, and that classical asthma, in which the lungs react by narrowing and the bronchi become inflamed when exposed to other irritants, dusts and pollens, is at the other extreme.

British researchers, on the other hand, tend to believe that the disease is the final result of damage caused by repeated chest infec-tions, and that it is quite separate from asthma, attacking a different group of people. The infections, they propose, arise because of smoke-induced damage to the bronchial lining. They admit that there are asthma-like responses in people with COPD, but that they arise from the diseased state and so are not due to true asthma. They point to the fact that the type of inflammation seen in sufferers of the disease differs from that in those with asthma.

Although the medical 'jury' is still pondering the evidence given by the two camps, there is at least agreement on one practical point: anti-asthmatic drugs can help greatly in the later stages of COPD (they will be described in Chapter 5).

Air pollution

In the 1950s, before the Clean Air Act in the UK put an end to the terrible winter 'smogs' in the cities, hospitals were, at times, filled to overflowing with people suffering chronic bronchitis. Most of them were, even when there was no smog, teetering on the edge of serious breathing difficulties. The smogs tipped them over this edge: the acid fumes from thousands of chimneys were the final insult to their already smoke-damaged lungs.

It was accepted then that industrial air pollution did not actually *cause* bronchitis in the first place, but that, once you had the disease, any form of pollution might make it worse. Medical students then were shown the healthy lungs from non-smokers who had lived in busy cities all their lives. They were contrasted with the lungs of smoking farmers, which were black, gritty and full of scars, despite the fact that their owners spent their lives in the fresh air.

We no longer have smogs in the UK, but the air pollution in our towns and cities is rising again, and this time it is much more insidious. It comes almost exclusively from motor vehicle exhausts and contains corrosive acid gases, such as the oxides of nitrogen and sulphur.

The work of Professor David Bates, of the University of British Columbia, and Dr Joel Schwartz, of the US Government's Environmental Protection Agency, suggested that such pollution will be much worse, in the long run, than the smog damage of the past. In the 1950s, Professor Bates was working in London's St Bartholomew's Hospital at the height of the smogs. At that time, the beds were full, patients lay wheezing in corridors, and patients were dying in ambulances on their way to hospital.

In the 1990s, Professor Bates and Dr Schwartz stressed that the patterns of deaths due to lung disease had risen to the level they were at in 1952. They blamed not the heavy black soot that caused the high incidence of lung disease in the 1950s by blocking the small bronchi, but much finer particles, called 'PM10s', from vehicle exhausts.

'PM10' stands for 'particulate matter less than 10 microns (10 thousandths of a millimetre) in diameter'. The smallest PM10s (less than 2.5 microns across) can enter the smallest bronchioles, and even the alveoli, and stick there. They may carry damaging chemicals such as acids on their surfaces. Indeed, more than 80 different chemicals have been identified as being 'stuck to' PM10s. The British Government's air monitoring station at the Warren Spring Laboratory in Stevenage, Hertfordshire, showed that PM10 concentrations in nine British cities regularly rose above acceptable levels. Professor Bates believed that in December 1991, before such monitors were in place, London levels of PM10s were six to eight times higher than the official American safety level of 150 micrograms of PM10s per cubic metre of air.

Dr Schwartz goes further. His studies suggest that there are *no* safe lower levels of PM10s, and that for every increase of PM10s of 10 micrograms per cubic metre of air, the death rate from lung disease rises by 1 per cent. He estimates that 60 thousand American citizens and 10 thousand people in England and Wales die directly because of vehicle exhaust pollution every year.

The problem with modern vehicle exhaust pollution, unlike the old smogs, is that we cannot see it (the particles do not make the lungs black and gritty), and we do not feel its effect in our lungs. We can smell it, though, and its smell is certainly present in every busy town. There is good evidence from the air monitoring team in St Mary's Hospital, London, that it has already endangered the lungs of the present generation of schoolchildren and young adults.

The St Mary's group was concerned, primarily, with pollen counts and hay fever. It noted that hay fever and asthma cases had risen steeply, despite falling pollen counts. The proportion of British schoolchildren with asthma rose from around 8 per cent to 15 per cent between 1960 and 1990. The figures for hay fever in young adults also doubled. In exactly the same period, pollen counts fell as green fields were taken over for building. For example, a third of all the grasslands in the Home Counties around the outskirts of London was built on between 1961 and 1991 – a loss of 300 thousand green acres.

There had to be an explanation – other than pollen allergy – for the soaring asthma and hay fever figures. The St Mary's team had no doubt what it is. They found that acid gases in the air alter pollen granules to make them more active as allergens. This helps explain the rise in hay fever cases. In the same 30 years, air pollution in the form of vehicle exhaust gases rose as steeply as, and in parallel with, the rising asthma and hay fever figures. Air pollution counts correlate closely with the numbers of admissions of people with breathing difficulties (which include those with asthma and acute bronchitis) to hospitals. On days of heavy traffic, there are many more admissions than usual.

Such figures have made the researchers think again about the relationship between air pollution and COPD. They reason that if rising levels of vehicle exhaust gases in the air can increase the numbers of people who suffer from hay fever and asthma, then they may well increase the numbers of cases of chronic bronchitis, too. The only difference from hay fever and asthma (in which the nose and lungs react immediately to the pollution) is that it will take much longer to identify the new bronchitis cases as the obvious symptoms only arise years after the first damage is done to the bronchi.

Current medical thinking in the UK still holds that most cases of chronic bronchitis are caused by smoking, but it is predicted that if air pollution from vehicle exhausts is allowed to continue, many more cases, even in non-smokers, may occur in the future. The medical message about pollution is only beginning to be heard by the car manufacturers and politicians. Let us hope that they take action soon to clean up the air in our towns and cities.

The lesson for anyone with COPD, however, is to keep well away from traffic-congested town centres or motorway jams. Urban air is becoming increasingly lethal, year by year.

Inherited COPD

A very small number of people with the disease (under 1 per cent) inherit it. They have a deficiency in their ability to make a substance called alpha-1 protease inhibitor or alpha-1 antitrypsin. This results in the breakdown of the structures of the alveoli, producing a gradually worsening emphysema during their later childhood and early adult lives. Their main symptom is a slowly increasing breathlessness.

Until recently, the only way to treat people with this type of COPD was to give transfusions or aerosol sprays of purified alpha-1 antitrypsin, prepared from human plasma taken from blood donors. As it took hundreds of units of blood to make just one dose of alpha-1 antitrypsin, and sufferers needed one transfusion per month, this was not practical.

Researchers in Edinburgh used genetic engineering to produce sheep that give human alpha-1 antitrypsin in their milk, and this is now supplying most of the British requirements for it. Patients using it are doing very well.

Work-related COPD

People whose jobs or hobbies expose them to dusts develop this disease more readily than does the rest of the population. It takes one of two forms: 'pneumoconiosis' and 'extrinsic allergic alveolitis'.

Pneumoconiosis

The commonest form of pneumoconiosis occurs in miners. In its simplest, uncomplicated form, pneumoconiosis rarely causes serious coughing or breathlessness, and once the exposure to coal stops, the lungs remain reasonably healthy. However, if the miner is also a smoker, then the combination of dust and smoke can cause extremely severe disease, with rapid deterioration of the lungs caused by extensive scarring, or 'fibrosis'.

Whether or not a miner develops pneumoconiosis depends on how much dust he is exposed to in his lifetime, and on the type of coal he has mined. Highly combustible coal, like the anthracite mined in South Wales, is more likely to cause chest disease than the usual 'steam' coals mined elsewhere. The highest risk to miners is coal that contains around 10 per cent quartz as this leads to particles of both coal and silica being deposited in the lungs.

Silicosis Unlike simple coal miners' pneumoconiosis, silicosis tends to progress, and can continue to worsen even after the exposure to the dust has stopped. Today, only around 100 people a year in the UK are diagnosed as having silicosis, a massive drop in numbers that reflects the falling numbers of people working, not just in mines, but in iron foundries, potteries and slate quarries, where silica dust has always been a health hazard. Cases are more likely to arise now in those who work in the fields of stonemasonry, metal mining, granite quarrying, tunnelling and coalmining where rock, as well as coal, must be cut. Sadly, according to Professor Anthony Seaton, former Professor of Environmental and Occupational Medicine at the University of Aberdeen, silicosis may again be on the rise as industry relaxes its measures regarding the control of dust in order to ensure greater productivity. The current British standard for the air breathed by people in mining and quarrying is 0.1 milligram of breathable (that is, very small) quartz particles in a cubic metre of air. Dust levels should be kept below this level in every workplace. Workers should also wear respirators as an extra measure, but they are not to be used as a substitute for dust control.

Among other dust-induced diseases, foundry work or welding can give rise to 'siderosis', which is when particles of iron work their way into the lungs. They are relatively benign, rarely giving rise to progressive COPD. People who mine china clay, shale or iron ore can suffer, respectively, from kaolin, shale or 'haematite' pneumoconiosis. Other occupations that can cause workers to have dusty lungs include tin refining and polyvinylchloride manufacture.

Asbestosis The most publicized of all the pneumoconioses is asbestosis. Asbestos is a form of fibrous silicate that is resistant to heat and to rotting, so it has been used widely in building construction for over a century. Its history goes back much further: it is said that the lamp wicks used by the vestal virgins in Roman times were made of asbestos.

The link between asbestos and lung disease, however, was only made in the 1950s, but legislation to protect against it (in the 1960s) has not prevented around thirty thousand people in the UK from being exposed to it to a significant degree. Cases of cancer due to the presence of asbestos in the lungs have been highlighted in the media, so that it has become the 'bogey' material for many pressure groups. Insurance claims for compensation against asbestos exposure in the USA were largely responsible for the huge losses made by Lloyds names from 1989 onwards and will continue to be so for years to come.

Looked at calmly, the media's fears about asbestos have been overstated. Asbestos occurs in two main forms: 'serpentine', or white, asbestos accounts for more than 95 per cent of all asbestos production, and is not particularly dangerous; 'amphibole' asbestos, which includes the brown or blue forms, is more likely to cause long-term lung disease.

The risk of disease after breathing in asbestos depends on how long you have been exposed to it and how heavily the air has been polluted with the asbestos dust. Dr Deborah Yates, a specialist in pneumoconiosis and allied diseases, reviewed the evidence against asbestos. Short fibres of asbestos (as would be yielded by white asbestos) are 'relatively harmless', she wrote in *Medicine International* in 1991. She added:

> Asbestos spraying and lagging produced the highest concentration of airborne fibres, with fewer fibres being produced by the sawing of asbestos-containing products. Fibre counts in buildings with disintegrating asbestos insulation are lower than fibre counts in city air, and the risks seem to have been exaggerated. Fibre levels are higher after removal of asbestos, even when carried out under stringent safety precautions. Asbestos bodies (particles of asbestos in the lung) are present in the lungs of every city dweller.

Asbestosis is a progressive scarring (fibrosis) of the lungs and this causes breathlessness, often with a dry cough. Some sufferers also complain of chest 'tightness' and feel that they cannot take a deep breath. In the later stages, chest infections are common, and the heart can begin to fail. Treatment is the same as for COPD due to smoking, which will be described in a later chapter. As with all pneumoconioses, asbestosis is made much worse, and progresses much faster towards heart failure, in a smoker, so it is essential in such cases for the sufferer to stop smoking. Also, asbestosis and smoking together multiplies the person's risk of lung cancer – an even more powerful reason to stop.

All these conditions should pass into history as regulations about safety at work should now make it impossible to inhale such dusts. In any dusty environment the law requires that there are regular measurements of fibres and particles in the air and all people working in a dusty atmosphere must wear positive pressure respirators. There are signs that this is happening, at least where there is a danger of conditions such as asbestosis. In the UK, only around 200 new cases of asbestosis are diagnosed each year, and almost all are men in their sixties or older who were laggers, dockyard workers or asbestos factory workers before 1969.

If you think your lung problem may have been caused by exposure to dust at work, then you should ask your doctor to refer you to a lung specialist for assessment. A straightforward chest X-ray of a pneumoconiosis sufferer shows a host of small, irregularly shaped shadows – in effect, the particles of dust – that are not seen in other forms of COPD. The International Labour Organisation has classified a series of X-rays in order of severity and comparing these standard X-rays with your own can help in any legal argument for compensation. The hospital doctor in charge of your case will have access to the ILO standard X-rays and can help to make the comparison.

If a diagnosis of occupational lung disease has been made, you can seek compensation in the UK either through the legal system or through a government scheme that gives a pension for life to proven sufferers of 'prescribed diseases'. Application forms (NI2, NI3, NI6 and NI237) can be obtained from the Department for Work and Pensions (for contact details, see page 104). Other countries have similar schemes. Advice on claims for asbestos-related diseases is offered by the Department for Work and Pensions.

Farmer's lung and other related problems – chronic extrinsic allergic alveolitis

The history of this condition dates from 1932, when the illness now known as 'farmer's lung' was first described. The only symptom of this chronic condition (it sometimes causes an acute asthma-like illness) is a gradual awareness of increasing breathlessness when engaging in physical activity. There may or may not be a cough, and the chest does not sound 'crackly' as in some COPD cases.

There is often no acute illness and the breathlessness may take years before it becomes so severe as to be a social drawback. However, this itself can be a disadvantage, as the diagnosis (which is made from the chest X-ray), can sometimes be delayed to a point at which recovery to a state of normal breathing is unlikely.

Farmer's lung is just one of many types of chronic lung disease arising from the inhalation of 'organic' dusts, that is, dusts from living organisms or chemical complexes, in the air. Table 1 shows how many of these disease-provoking dusts have been identified to date, and the occupations and hobbies that put people at risk. Most of these illnesses are caused by micro-organisms such as bacteria and moulds, and some originate from animals, while others come from plants and a few from chemicals.

All these forms of dust-induced disease are caused by inflammation (to be exact, an allergic reaction) within the alveoli, not the bronchi, which explains the relative absence of cough and mucus, which are usually symptoms of bronchitis. Most occur because the stored material has become contaminated by micro-organisms and then dried out, so that when it is moved (for example hay in a barn, or grain in a silo) the air is filled with clouds of microscopic particles to which the lung is highly sensitive. So, farmer's lung, for example, is not initiated at harvest time, but perhaps months or years later, when the stored material is moved or used. Thus, it is at these times that people should be very careful to protect their lungs.

Often, there is a 'cocktail' of micro-organisms in the air – moulds and bacteria together – that cause the illness. This is particularly the case in the huge industrial humidifiers installed in textile factories, which can harbour a host of lung disease-provoking organisms. In the USA it is estimated that between 15 and 52 per cent of the population exposed to industrial humidifiers have humidifier lung.

Table 1 The causes of alveolitis – farmer's lung and similar diseases

Causes	Source	Name of lung disease
Bacteria and moulds	Paper mill pulp	Wood pulp worker's lung
	Whisky maltings	Malt worker's lung
	Vegetable compost	Farmer's/gardener's lung
	Dog bedding	Dog house disease
	Sewage	Sewage worker's lung
	Maple	Maple stripper's lung
	Puffballs	Lycoperdonosis
	Paprika	Paprika splitter's lung
	Cheese	Cheese washer's lung
	Cork	Suberosis
	Horse barn straw	Stable disease
	Hay/straw/grain/ compost	Farmer's lung
	Mushroom compost	Mushroom worker's lung
	Air conditioners	Humidifier lung
	Saunas	Sauna taker's lung
Animals:		
Mites	Grain dust	Granary lung
Birds	Bloom/excreta	Bird fancier's lung
Fish	Fish meal	Fish meal worker's lung
Mammals	Fur	Furrier's lung
Rodents	Urine	Laboratory worker's lung
Plants:		
Wood	Sawdust	Woodworker's lung
Chemicals:		
Bordeaux mixture	Vineyards	Vineyard sprayer's lung
Cobalt	Tungsten carbide grinding	
Formaldehyde	Laboratory	
Pyrethrum	Insecticide spray	
Diisocyanates	Plastics industry	
Trimellitic anhydride	Plastics industry	

In the UK, 1 to 2 per cent of people are farmers. In regions where there is heavy rainfall and farm produce is stored traditionally without using drying machines, 10 per cent of the farmers have some degree of farmer's lung. This is more than ten times the rate found in farmers using modern storage and drying facilities. Bird fancier's lung used to be common in the UK, where in the 1990s around 12 per cent of households had pet budgerigars. It is still a problem for those who keep homing pigeons, and remains the commonest form of dust-induced chronic lung disease in the UK. Estimates of bird fancier's lung range from less than 1 per cent to 21 per cent of the pigeon-keeping population.

No doubt you will now be beginning to realize why your doctor, when he or she hears about your cough and breathlessness, asks you so many questions about your work and home environment, present and past. You will also understand why they may order so many investigations to find out the cause. There is often much more to a 'simple' cough than at first seems possible.

The next chapter describes the typical course of COPD and the tests doctors order to find the cause. The test results are important, because the choice of treatment largely depends on them.

3

The course of COPD: tests and exercise

The progress of COPD

Most adults who smoke and have chronic simple bronchitis see themselves as normal. The only symptoms may be a constant need to clear the throat and to swallow mucus that has appeared in the back of the mouth. They ignore their early morning cough, just after waking, thinking that everyone does it. However, the production of as little as 2 millilitres of phlegm per day is abnormal and is likely to lead to the need to cough throughout the day.

Over the years, the cough very gradually worsens. The phlegm, at first, is just clear mucus, perhaps flecked with tiny black dots from the smoke. Occasionally, the spit is yellow or green and the cough is complicated by bouts of breathlessness. These are signs of infection. The coloured sputum may persist beyond the acute illness as the infection grumbles on, quietly, in the bronchi.

Then comes the crunch, the illness that finally convinces the smoker that there is something seriously wrong with their chest. After many years of coughing, but not much else, the first really disabling chest infection hits. It usually happens in winter and keeps the sufferer away from work for a week or more. The infection is often accompanied, or followed, by the first attacks of breathlessness.

From then on, the breathlessness worsens, very gradually. At first, it is just more noticeable with fairly severe exertion. Then it starts to interfere with sports activities and slowly it begins to impinge on normal everyday actions. This breathlessness is a sign that the smaller airways are narrowing and blocking with inflammation and mucus, and that emphysema may have started. For the first time, there may be wheezing.

Sometimes an infection leaves the chest much worse than before, making the coughing more persistent and the breathlessness more severe, and takes much longer to clear, perhaps never completely returning to normal. By this time it is getting difficult to breathe out fully, so that the chest always seems to be expanded, even when a special effort is made to empty the lungs of air. The neck and shoulder muscles are used more to try to force more air into and out of the chest, even at rest.

Later still, as even the most strenuous efforts fail to get enough oxygen into the lungs, the heart begins to feel the strain. The face becomes tinged with blue and bloated, the eyes become red and swollen, and the chest barrel-shaped, out of proportion with the rest of the body. Each breath is a struggle.

The aim of all treatment for COPD is to prevent this final stage or at least postpone it for many years. The following chapters describe how this can be done. First, however, anyone with suspected COPD needs to have the extent of their disease assessed by tests.

Who gets chronic lung disease?

Chronic bronchitis and emphysema affects men and women alike. The vast majority of sufferers are smokers, and the severity of the illness – how much you cough, how much sputum you produce, how breathless you are on how little exertion, and how rapidly your breathing deteriorates – depends directly on how many cigarettes you smoke per day. Women's lungs seem to be more sensitive than men's to the effects of smoke, so that 10 cigarettes a day for a woman is equivalent to around 20 a day for men. Severe symptoms usually start in middle age, say in the thirties for heavy smokers, and late forties for those who smoke under a pack a day.

A small number of non-smokers develop COPD. They have usually inherited a problem, either with their cilia or their ability to produce normal mucus, or they have had a severe lung infection in infancy or childhood (see Chapter 2).

Examining the lungs

If COPD is suspected, your doctor will spend some time watching you breathe, at rest, noting how well your chest expands and, particularly, how deeply you can breathe *out*. This is because as the disease progresses, it is more and more difficult to expel air from the lungs, so that the chest seems to be constantly expanded. Less than 5 centimetres (2 inches) of chest expansion between breathing in and out suggests that the COPD needs special care.

The sounds heard through the stethoscope while you breathe in and out tell the doctor where the air flow is normal and where it is disturbed. However, they may *sound* normal even in cases of advanced bronchitis. This contrasts strongly with the wheeze heard on breathing out in someone with asthma. Over areas of bronchiectasis, very prominent 'crackles' can be heard on breathing out and in. In emphysema, the breath sounds are fainter than normal.

Chest X-rays, like the breath sounds, are not particularly helpful in most cases of bronchitis, but they do show areas of bronchiectasis. They show streaks and spots of dust in the lungs of people with dust-linked diseases. In the later stages of COPD, the heart enlarges in response to the strain, and this, of course, can be seen on an X-ray.

However, neither listening to, nor X-raying, the chest gives any real idea of how well the lungs are working. This can only be assessed by the technique of spirometry. For this you will be asked to take part in several breathing tests.

Breathing tests

Peak flow, or PF, levels

The first and simplest breathing test, which you may be asked to do daily at home, is the 'peak flow', or PF. The PF meter measures how hard and how fast you can blow out after the deepest possible breath. A normal adult has PF levels of 500–600 litres per minute. In early bronchitis it may be near normal for many years; later it falls slowly (when it falls below 300–350 litres, you need help).

Daily PF measurements are most useful when an element of wheezing is involved in the illness. Wheezing is the classic symptom of asthma, which is caused by the inflammation of the bronchi and spasm of the muscles in the bronchial wall that occur during an attack, resulting in an extreme narrowing of the bronchi. The wheezing, a high-pitched whistle-like sound on breathing out, is the result of trying to force air *out* from over-inflated alveoli through narrowed bronchi with thickened walls. For asthma sufferers, steroid inhalers are given to suppress the inflammation and 'bronchodilator' inhalers to widen the bronchi, and the results of using them can be seen almost immediately – the wheezing stops and there is a steep rise in the PF level.

In asthma attacks, PF levels can dip well below 300 litres, and levels around 200 litres in an adult can be life-threatening. In the UK, all those who need to have their asthma controlled with medication have their own PF meters and record their PF level every day. A gradual drop in their PF level means an attack of acute asthma may be imminent, so they increase their inhaler doses accordingly.

In COPD, the changes in PF levels are rarely as acute or as severe as they are in those who have asthma. However, almost everyone with COPD eventually develops some degree of wheezing, so that they, too, can benefit from anti-asthma inhaler treatment. Many people with COPD are therefore asked to record their PF levels daily, and to manage their wheezing accordingly.

Other tests

Three other spirometry measurements are more relevant than PF levels to people with COPD. They are:

- Forced Expiratory Volume in One Second (FEV1)
- Slow Vital Capacity (SVC)
- Forced Vital Capacity (FVC).

To perform these tests, you breathe air through a tube into a drum, which rises and falls with the air entering and leaving. The volume of air you breathe is recorded on computer.

The Forced Expiratory Volume in One Second measurement   This is the maximum amount of air you can blow out of your lungs in one second after taking a deep breath. This amount is reduced when there is narrowing of both large and small bronchi, as is the case with longstanding bronchitis.

The Slow Vital Capacity measurement This is the volume of air being breathed in and out with each breath when the person is relaxed.

The Forced Vital Capacity measurement This is the same volume that is measured during a Slow Vital Capacity test, but this time it is measured when the person is breathing as hard and fast as possible.

In cases of emphysema, the Forced Vital Capacity measurement is often lower than the Slow Vital Capacity one because the lung's ability to 'recoil' (its elasticity) is reduced. The effort of trying to breathe out forcibly closes off the smaller airways and traps air in the alveoli. COPD patients with differences between these two measurements have to learn how to control their breathing correctly, especially with exercise.

Exercise tolerance

The ability to exercise is often a more sensitive test of how well your lungs are doing than spirometry, and is, of course, much more relevant to your quality of life. The one most often used is the six-minute walk test, which measures the distance you can walk on the flat in six minutes, inclusive of stops for rest. Walk tests like this are used to assess improvement and deterioration of COPD in response to treatment or after infections. Walk test results can vary from day to day, so they should be interpreted with caution by someone with experience in this area.

Many general practitioners ask their patients to do the 'lamp-post' test, asking how many lamp-posts they can pass without stopping for breath, say, on the way to the surgery or shops. Lamp-post tests can be a good rough guide to progress when the 'results' are noted over a period of several months.

The important point about exercise tolerance testing is that it gives you some idea of the improvements you can make in your breathing yourself, quite apart from any treatment you may receive from your doctor.

Exercise is a vital part of your own long-term management of the disease. Many people with COPD, and many of their carers, are frightened by the breathlessness that comes with exertion, thinking that it may cause further damage to the lungs, but this is not so. Exercising until you are in a state of breathlessness is actually *good* for the lungs, not bad, and people with COPD should be encouraged to do it – if possible, daily.

How exercise can help you breathe more easily

Even if you are breathless while resting, there are always exercises to do that can help you breathe more easily.

Gentle, normal breathing uses the lower half of the chest. If you have COPD, however, you may be in the habit of using the upper chest to the virtual exclusion of the lower chest. This takes much more effort than normal breathing and can exhaust you sooner.

To change back to normal breathing, first, sit down, ensuring that your back is well supported. Make sure that, during the exercise, you do *not* hold your breath at any time, as this can cause you to worry or even panic.

Now, breathe out gently while consciously relaxing your shoulders and upper chest. When you feel you are ready, slowly breathe in, but keep your upper chest relaxed. You should feel your lower ribs and your upper abdomen opening out as the air enters your chest – a sensation like breathing around the waist. If you wish, put your hands on your lower ribs and upper abdomen as you do this to feel what you are doing, or you can watch the movement in a mirror. Continue for 10 minutes or more, keeping the breathing rhythm steady and smooth, so that it becomes automatic.

You may find that 'pursed lip' breathing is a good aid to controlling the rate and depth of your breathing. In this exercise, you breathe in slowly and deeply through the nose, then breathe out equally slowly through pursed lips. 'Counted breathing' can help in the same way. Count 'one, two' in your head while breathing in and 'three, four' while breathing out. Some find counting 'three, four, five' when breathing out is even better. When you climb stairs, count two steps for breathing in and three, four steps for breathing out.

'Huffing', or active cycle breathing

Active cycle breathing is a routine that helps people to clear their phlegm. It starts with relaxed, controlled breathing, then this is followed by deep breathing and a forced expiration or 'huff'.

The relaxed breathing, using the lower chest muscles, described above, prevents you 'tightening up' during the exercise and from becoming dizzy as a result of taking too many deep breaths. Throughout the cycle, keep using the lower rib and abdominal muscles.

Once your breathing is relaxed and comfortable, begin to take deep breaths. Concentrate on breathing in; breathing out will take care of itself. By taking deep breaths, you are driving air into the alveoli, beyond the collections of mucus.

After five deep breaths, return to the initial 'relaxed' breathing. When the relaxed pattern is settled, try a 'huff'.

To huff, take a medium breath, then squeeze all the air out of your chest by tightening your stomach muscles. Do not make a loud noise at the back of your throat as that means that the huff is not deep enough in your chest. If the huff makes you cough, make the cough short or your chest will tighten up. Huffing will help to move sputum and short coughs will help to bring it up.

Blowing up balloons

As a break from huffing, you may like to try balloon blowing. Dr Bernard Leahy, a consultant chest physician in Manchester, found that his patients with bronchitis and emphysema reported fewer episodes of breathlessness and that they felt much better generally after blowing up children's balloons every day.

He asked 22 of his patients with COPD to perform the six-minute walk test (see page 31). He measured how far they could walk in six minutes, including stops for rests. He then split them into two groups of 11, and asked them to record each period of breathlessness they experienced during the next eight weeks. One group, however, also had to blow up a balloon 20 times each evening.

When the walking test was repeated at the end of this eight-week period, the balloon-blowers improved their distance by an average of 15 per cent. The others experienced no change in their condition.

My own patients who have tried this 'treatment' have found it odd at first, but have reported later that it has 'loosened up' their chests and helped them to cough out phlegm. It seems to help both those with bronchitis and emphysema and has resulted in improvements in their lung test results.

Organizing your exercise

Start your exercise programme slowly, going just a little further each day. Your doctor and/or physiotherapist will set your goals for you (everyone is different). When you walk, let your arms hang loosely by your sides, with your shoulders and chest relaxed. Plan ahead to bring in stairs and uphill slopes if you can. Stairs give variety and more effective exercise. Keep in mind that exercise that makes you breathless is *not* harmful and that you are in control. If your breathlessness becomes distressing, however, then simply stopping and relaxing for a few minutes will return you to normal.

Relaxation

Relaxation is an essential in all forms of exercise. To relax between periods of exercise, always make sure that you are comfortable. Listen to soothing music: choose music that you like. My own preference is for soft, slow classical rhythms, but whether your taste is classical, country or something else, it should be music you can dream to! Then, relax every group of muscles in the body, in turn.

Most relaxation exercises start at the toes, then work their way up through the feet, the ankles, calves, thighs, trunk, back and chest muscles, shoulders, arms, wrists and fingers, before finishing with the neck, facial and scalp muscles. If you can take time to do this for a few minutes a day, it will help you to tackle your exercises more effectively.

You may like to take your relaxation further, and using the Alexander Technique is an excellent way to do this. F. M. Alexander was a former Australian actor who developed the technique and then taught his form of relaxation to others at the end of the nineteenth century. His exercises are still relevant today.

His basic philosophy was that we perform many of our everyday actions, such as sitting and walking, wrongly, and that this puts strains on our bodies. F. M. Alexander showed that the way we sit and stand can affect the way we breathe. We tend to slump in upon ourselves, bending our backs and compressing our ribcages inwards, onto our lungs. This reduces the amount of air we can breathe in. To compensate for this, we tend to hold ourselves upright from the shoulders, compressing our chests further and putting strain on our backs. If we have a chronic lung condition as well as this kind of bad posture, the anxiety and tension we feel are multiplied.

The Alexander Technique helps people to relax and breathe more naturally. It is taught on an individual basis, with the Alexander practitioner helping the person to develop an understanding of how their routine posture and muscle use is wrong and how to correct it. Lessons are given by qualified Alexander instructors. They study for three years at an approved training school – often in an instructor's home. Some instructors visit patients, and sessions take from 45 minutes to an hour. Most people find three to four lessons are beneficial and that they have then learned enough to practise the techniques that help with their particular difficulties on their own. If you would like to know more, contact the Society of Teachers of the Alexander Technique at the address given on page 105.

Go for it!

If you think that all this exercise is not for you, think again. The British Lung Foundation's newsletter *Breathing Space* (more about the Foundation in Chapter 8), records some real success stories. The people mentioned have kindly given their permission for me to repeat them here.

One of these is the story of David Frater. While in hospital with a collapsed lung (a complication of his emphysema), he realized that his physiotherapist's advice on deep breathing was the same as his own technique for bagpiping. So he took up the pipes again. He has improved his PF levels from around 100 to 250 litres (176 to 440 pints), and is keeping them there! He practises his 'physiotherapy' three times a week for 15 to 20 minutes at a time.

Then there is Sheila Moss. She has McLeod's syndrome, an inherited form of emphysema. She celebrated her fiftieth birthday by deciding to do something about her 'lifetime of breathlessness'. She gradually built up the amount of exercise she did and whereas she used to become breathless after a few yards, she can now *run* a third of a mile, and she finished a sponsored walk over hilly country in under two and a half hours. Her ambition is to run a mile, and she says that she has run half a mile – downhill!

She feels healthier and fitter than she has ever done, and her doctor confirms that her lung tests have improved from 35 per cent of normal to 60 per cent. She advises other people with the condition to 'go for it'.

Even if your disease is crippling by any standards, this need not exclude you from taking part in sport.

For example, Margaret Lloyd-Roberts has a six-year-long career (so far) as cox to a rowing club. Margaret has Kartagener's syndrome (see page 14), and has both cilia dyskinesia (in which the cilia cannot transport mucus up towards the throat) and bronchiectasis.

When we asked her if her lung condition deterred her, she replied:

'All the fresh air is ideal. A standard boat is 60 feet long and in order to make my voice carry I have to take deep breaths and control my breathing. Occasionally I have a chance to row, which I enjoy, and, of course, that really is a good rhythmic exercise for the chest and lungs. I also attend training sessions. I do about one press up to every five of theirs and drop out when I've had enough. Everyone is very encouraging and concerned for my wellbeing. Training sessions are run by a member who is a physiotherapist, so it couldn't be better.'

She added:

'I've found a sport that suits me. I can take part without having a great deal to do physically. The camaraderie is great. I'm treated very much as one of the crew. I have the blessing of my GP, who actually used to be a cox himself, provided that I wrap up warm. Above all it means that my lung condition doesn't get me down.'

If you are thinking 'These examples are all very well, but my lungs are too far gone even to contemplate moving out of the house', think again.

Don Blakey is a good example of someone who just will not give up. He is 80, has had emphysema for 12 years, and can be seen each summer driving the 670 miles from the French channel ports to the foothills of the Pyrenees, where he and his wife Jackie spend their holidays. This is not unusual, you may think, until you learn that he wears his oxygen-delivering nebulizer mask as he drives! The plug fits into the car cigar lighter socket.

Of course, Don and Jackie do have to plan their journey carefully, to include the stop-over point in France where they are well known. The ferry company gives them reduced fares and the ship's doctor arranges for Don to use his nebulizer while he is travelling. All eventualities, therefore, are foreseen.

Don's adventures, though, go beyond merely driving long distances. Watching someone gliding a few years ago, he ended up having a go himself, even taking the controls at one point!

The lessons to be learned from all these people – and every family doctor could add other examples – is that while there is breath, there is hope. *Do* keep on going, because the effort you make can keep your lungs as healthy as they can be. Doctors and physiotherapists can do much to help, but the real drive to continue has to come from within *you*. Hopefully, these examples of the triumphs of people with very severe lung disease will prompt you to be all you can be, too.

Eating wisely

It may seem odd in a book about chest disease to include a section on eating, but it is, in fact, very appropriate. If you have lung disease it is best to be within 6.3 kilograms (1 stone) of the correct weight for your height.

If you are overweight, then lose the excess slowly. Do not go on a crash diet, but aim instead to lose about 1 kilogram (2 pounds) a month. Combine a sensible, low-calorie diet (of not less than 1000 calories per day) with as much regular exercise as you can manage. Also, limit your alcohol intake; grill rather than fry food; eat plenty of vegetables and fruit; and take time over your meals.

About one in three people with COPD are underweight rather than obese. Often the exertion of eating even a medium meal makes them too breathless, so they do not take in enough food for their energy needs. If this describes you, or even if your weight is normal, there are ways to improve your eating habits. Meals *can* become a pleasure again, rather than a chore, and they will not make you nearly so breathless if you adhere to the following advice.

- *Eat smaller meals more often.* Six small meals a day make you less breathless than three larger ones. If chewing tires you out, liquidize the food.
- *Eat high-energy foods.* Small quantities of food high in starch, such as chocolate biscuits, are easier to digest and give much more energy for a much smaller bulk in the stomach than, for example, a large salad.
- *Avoid 'gassy' foods.* When your COPD is giving problems, avoid foods that form gas in the bowel, as the distension in the abdomen presses up against the diaphragm, compressing the space for the lungs. This may make your breathlessness even worse. Among the worst offenders are apples, melons, Brussels sprouts, peas and beans, turnips, cabbage, corn and cucumber.
- *Consume liquids, rather than solids.* Drinking uses up less energy than chewing, so, during bad periods, replace several of your six meals a day with high-energy drinks, such as high-protein milk shakes. Home-made liquidized foods are excellent, as are commercial products such as Complan or instant soups. Some patients qualify for free prescriptions of liquid foods, but you need to discuss whether or not you do with your doctor.
- *Avoid hard, dry foods.* Any foods, like crackers, that need considerable chewing can sap your energy, so avoid them. Choose instead softer foods, such as fruit, and take sauces or custard with your food to make them easier to chew.
- *Clean your mouth before meals.* Inhaled or nebulized drugs often leave a bad taste in the mouth that can spoil your appetite. You can remove it, and regain your appetite, by cleaning your teeth, using a mouthwash or chewing gum. Choose whichever of these suits you best.

If you have particular problems with your weight, your doctor may well ask you to take advice from a dietitian colleague. Making changes in your eating habits need not mean that food becomes boring. The British Heart Foundation has produced a pamphlet entitled *Eating Well* (to obtain a copy you can write to the Foundation at the address given on page 103). Although it is meant for heart patients and people wishing to avoid or prevent heart disease, it is entirely appropriate for people with lung trouble, too.

Once you have reached your ideal weight, try to stay at that weight by continuing with your healthy eating regimen and by regularly exercising up to your limit. If you can do this, you have done all you can to help yourself, bar one thing. That is stopping smoking. If you are already a non-smoker, you can miss out the next chapter, but if you smoke, it is the most important one in the book for you. By the time you have read it, if you are *still* determined to continue smoking, then there is no point in reading further. There is nothing anyone can do for you.

4

Stopping smoking

What happens when I smoke?

If you have chest disease and you smoke, you are either mad or tired of life. Even for the healthy, smoking is a stupid habit with nothing to recommend it. It is not only the main cause of COPD, it also puts you at risk of heart attacks, and cancers of the lungs, kidneys and bladder. It destroys the delicate blood vessels in your legs, so that you can be left with gangrene and the possibility of amputations being required. It raises your blood pressure, making you more susceptible to strokes. Further, just because you already have COPD, this does not mean that you cannot develop all these other conditions, too!

Smoking gives people a sallow, unhealthy look and wrinkles. By the time they are 40, women smokers look 10 years older than their non-smoking sisters. By 60 many are already dead. Records of COPD, lung cancer and heart attacks, given as causes of death and all directly due to smoking, show that they result in far more early deaths in women than anything else.

If you already have lung disease, continuing to smoke accelerates your progress towards lung failure. All smokers, by their mid thirties, even if they do not notice any symptoms of chest disease, show some deterioration in their spirometry tests (see pages 29–31). Their Forced Expiratory Volume in One Second levels are already lower than normal and, with each passing year, they deteriorate faster than the slow drop that normally occurs with age.

As long ago as 1977, Drs Charles Fletcher and Richard Peto drew attention in the *British Medical Journal* to how fast lungs deteriorate when people continue to smoke, and how the deterioration can be slowed simply by stopping. They showed, too, that it is never too late to stop: smokers who stop at the age of 65 still derive benefit from breathing cleaner air. If you stop at 45, you can postpone the start of disability from COPD by around 20 years. If you stop at 65, you can still expect 4 extra years of reasonable life.

Virtually all adult smokers started their habit as teenagers, when they were too immature to think about its long-term consequences. If you are still a non-smoker by the time you are 20, it is odds on that you will remain so for the rest of your life. By this time you have learned sense!

Starting young is significant. In a study of British doctors carried out in the 1960s and 1970s, there were twice as many deaths from COPD among those who smoked more than 25 cigarettes a day than in those who smoked fewer than 15 per day, and deaths from this disease among the non-smokers were virtually nil. The pipe and cigar smokers had death rates between the non-smokers and those who daily smoked fewer than 15 cigarettes. Further, the earlier they started to smoke, the worse were their chances of dying early from COPD.

For most people who have COPD, it was that first decision to light up as teenagers that led to the lung problem they have today. If this describes you, today is the day to reverse that decision. You surely now have the maturity and common sense to do so.

If you need more persuasion, then the next few pages set out the arguments against smoking. Read them, please. I have found that when people sit down and think seriously about all these aspects of smoking, they almost always give up.

Your very first cigarette made you nauseous, dizzy and ill, as the poisons in the smoke entered your brain. New smokers have to be persuaded to continue by their tobacco-addicted friends (a sign of true addicts is that they want to persuade others to adopt their habit). Within days, the addiction takes hold. Now the smoker feels unwell without a cigarette – withdrawal symptoms take over from the initial unpleasant experience. From then on, it is downhill all the way. After a few years, the smoker will get through between 20 and 60 cigarettes a day.

To doctors like myself, who have had to comfort so many families in which smoking has directly led to the deaths of loved ones only in their forties and fifties, it is, frankly, incredible that anyone would wish to light up a single cigarette. To a smoker, ciga-rettes are more important than life itself.

How, exactly, does smoking harm the lungs? Among other noxious substances, tobacco smoke contains tiny sparks glowing at around 400° (752°F). They are far too small to feel and, in any case, because they bypass the nose (see page 4) and are sucked down directly into the chest, there are no nerves in the bronchial tree that are sensitive to them. It's estimated that for each puff of a cigarette, thousands of cilia are burned away. Smoke ten cigarettes a day for years and you can estimate how many of your precious cilia will be lost. They are replaced with fibrous scars.

These tiny burns are only the start of the damage. The smoke also contains tars – chemicals that corrode and damage the delicate, smooth lining of the whole bronchial tree. Cigarette tars contain more than a thousand different chemicals, several hundred of which are known to stimulate cancers. Ponder on that before you light up your next cigarette!

Thankfully, most cigarette smokers do not develop cancer, although enough of them do so to make this alone a good enough reason to stop. However, *all* cigarette smokers develop some degree of COPD, and the tars inhaled are always involved in its cause. They add to the burn damage by destroying the delicate ciliated cells, and the bronchi respond by increasing the number and activity of the goblet cells in an attempt to wash out the tars by producing more mucus. The attempt is in vain, because the cilia that would remove the excess fluid are either no longer there or cannot any more act in unison.

As if this were not bad enough, smoke also contains three other lung-destroying materials: particles of tobacco ash, nicotine and carbon monoxide gas. The ash acts like all the other dusts that can cause alveolar disease (see Table 1, page 25), an action thought to be responsible for around 98 per cent of all cases of emphysema. Nicotine is a powerful constrictor of blood vessels, so that the delicate balance between the alveolar surface and the blood flow through the lungs is disturbed. It also stimulates clotting of the blood in the capillaries, the smallest blood vessels in the lung into which the oxygen must pass. The net result is less oxygen exchange between incoming air and the blood circulation in the body.

The carbon monoxide in the smoke makes an already unfavourable state even worse. It, too, can cross over the membrane from alveoli to capillaries (see page 11), where it displaces oxygen from the blood and sticks there. The result is much poorer distribution of oxygen throughout the rest of the body – the brain and heart suffering the ill effects of this the most.

It is hard to imagine anything that the human mind could devise that would have as many harmful effects on the lungs and heart as smoking. It irritates and destroys the lungs, it causes both bronchitis *and* emphysema, it reduces the capacity of the blood to carry oxygen, it poisons the heart muscle (with carbon monoxide) and the brain (with nicotine and carbon monoxide), it narrows the coronary arteries (with nicotine) and promotes clotting inside them.

Imagine for a moment that cigarettes had just been discovered and that someone now wanted to try to bring them onto the market for the first time. No food or drugs authority anywhere in the world would allow this to happen. Their promoters might even be prosecuted for deliberately trying to damage human health.

Sadly, though, tobacco has been with us for hundreds of years, so it has escaped such governmental scrutiny. Also, governments make so much money from the taxes levied on it that few take steps to reduce its real impact on health. It is up to the individual to resist its advertiser's blandishments.

King James the Sixth of Scotland and First of England got it right when he wrote – over 400 years ago – that he found tobacco:

> Loathsome to the eye, hateful to the nose, harmful to the brain, dangerous to the lungs, and in the black stinking pit thereof nearest resembling the horrible Stygian smoke of the pit that is bottomless.

Believe King James and react appropriately. If even he does not completely convince you, consider the following facts about smoking:

- Smoking plays a main part in most deaths from heart disease, COPD, and lung cancer.
- Smokers are more than twice as likely to suffer a fatal heart attack

as non-smokers, the risk of this happening rising directly in proportion to the number of cigarettes smoked per day.

- Men younger than 45 who smoke 25 or more cigarettes a day
  have a 10 to 15 times greater chance of a fatal heart attack than
  non-smokers.
- In developed countries, such as the UK, a third of men die before
  they reach the retirement age of 65, and most of these deaths
  result from smoking-related disease, smoking being the major
  widow maker.
- 40 per cent of all heavy smokers die before their sixty-fifth
  birthday, and of the remaining 60 per cent, many are disabled
  by bronchitis, angina, heart failure or the need for leg amputations – all due to smoking.
- Only 10 per cent of smokers survive to 75 in good health; most
  non-smokers are healthy at that age.
- 40 per cent of all deaths from cancer in the UK are due to lung
  cancer (of 441 male British doctors who died of lung cancer, only
  7 had never smoked).
- Only 1 non-smoker in 60 develops lung cancer (even then, the
  cause may be passive smoke), while the figure for heavy smokers
  is 1 in 6.
- One non-smoker per day in the UK dies from lung cancer caused
  by passive smoking.
- Other smoking-related cancers include tumours of the tongue,
  throat, larynx, pancreas, kidney, bladder and cervix, with a third
  of *all* cancers being caused directly by smoking.

Perhaps I am beginning to persuade you to stop smoking. Good.
Doubtless, though, you will have heard, and probably used yourself, a host of excuses to avoid stopping. Doctors hear these all
the time from their patients. Here they are, together with my
counter-arguments. Do not let any of these excuses weaken your
resolve.

- *My uncle/father/grandfather smoked 20 a day and lived to 75.*
  We all know someone like that, but we forget all the many others
  who died long before their time. The chances are that you will be
  one of the many, not one of the rare lucky ones.

- *People who do not smoke also have lung disease.*
  True, but more than 98 per cent of all people who have serious COPD are smokers or ex-smokers, and for the few whose disease is inherited, smoking makes it much worse.

- *Moderation in everything is my rule; I only smoke moderately.*
  To assume this will save you is foolhardy to say the least. We do not accept moderation in lead poisoning, dangerous driving or violence. There is *no* lower safe limit to cigarette smoking; one a day is one too many.

- *I can cut down rather than stop.*
  You can, but it will not help. People who cut down usually take more puffs from each cigarette, leave a smaller butt, and end up with the same amount of carbon monoxide and nicotine in their bloodstream. The only answer is to stop completely.

- *I am just as likely to be run over in the road as to die from smoking.*
  In the UK, traffic causes 15 deaths a day. COPD causes 100, as do lung cancer and heart attacks, which is 20 times as many daily deaths. Of every 1000 young men who smoke, on average, 1 will be murdered, 6 will die on the roads and 250 will die before their time because they smoke.

- *I have to die of something.*
  I have always found that this is said by someone in good health. It is not said by anyone who has already developed a chronic illness, such as COPD or heart disease.

- *I do not want to be old, anyway.*
  We change our definition of 'old' as we grow older! We would all like to live a long time, but we do not want to be afflicted by the illnesses we see in the elderly. If we take care of ourselves on the way to old age we should enjoy it a lot more when we get there.

- *I will stop if my breathlessness/cough gets worse.*
  It has become progressively worse up to now, though! Do you want to wait until your first heart attack, or your first sign of lung cancer? Then it will be too late.

- *I will put on weight if I stop.*
  You probably will, but for most people with COPD this would not be a bad thing. Your appetite will return, and you will taste food again. Any weight you put on will come off again as you manage to exercise more. The health risks of being a bit over-weight are far less serious than those you will face if you keep on smoking.

- *I enjoy smoking and do not want to give up.*
  Are you sure? Is this not just an excuse because it sounds better than admitting you *cannot* stop? Is there *real* pleasure in smoking? Be honest with yourself.

- *Cigarettes settle my nerves. If I stopped I would have to take Valium.*
  Smoking is certainly a prop, like a baby's dummy. Its rituals – the packet, the lighter, the fondling of the cigarette, holding it in the mouth – all tend to be a substitute for boredom and even loneliness, but it solves nothing. It does not remove the causes of stress, and only worsens your long-term health prospects. If you already have the cough and breathlessness of COPD, each cigarette you light is a source of stress as it reminds you of the damage you are doing to your lungs, so you will *increase* your underlying anxiety, not reduce it.

- *I will change to a pipe or cigars – they are safer.*
  Lifelong pipe and cigar smokers are still ten times more likely to have COPD than non-smokers. Further, cigarette smokers who change to pipes or cigars do not reduce their chances of severe lung disease, probably because they continue to inhale.

- *I have smoked for 40 years. It's too late to give up.*
  It is *not* too late, whatever age you stop. Apart from postponing the onset of symptoms of COPD, stopping now will immediately reduce your risk of heart attacks and, if you can quit cigarettes for 15 years, you will reduce your chances of lung cancer by 80 per cent.

- *I wish I could stop. I have tried everything, but nothing has worked.*
  Stopping smoking is easy, if you *really* want to do it. Of course,

you must put some effort into it yourself and not expect someone else to do it for you. This means being motivated to do it. If you have not been motivated by the last few pages then you never will be!

Stopping smoking

Getting motivated

What motivates people to stop smoking varies from person to person, and from generation to generation.

Teenagers, for example, care little about long-term health risks. The health risks that will accrue to them in middle age, not to mention old age, are too remote to act as powerful motivation for them. They may even be *attracted* to the idea that smoking puts them in danger. If you want a teenager not to smoke, then concentrate on the way smoking makes them look and smell. Smoking *is* smelly and dirty. It also pollutes the environment and exploits poverty in the Global South to the benefit of big multinational business. These are very much the concerns of the younger generation. Pakistan, for example, uses 48 600 hectares (120 000 acres) and Brazil 202 500 hectares (500 000 acres) of fertile land to produce tobacco for the developed world's pleasure – at the expense of growing food for their poor. Even worse, the tobacco companies are vigorously promoting their wares to populations in the Global South, adding COPD and heart disease to their already huge burden of ill health. Find the teenager who wants to be party to this process?

For women in their younger adult years, appearance can be the best motivation to stop. Smoking ages people prematurely. Nicotine-induced changes in the skin circulation produce more wrinkles and a grey, pasty colour, rather than the normal, attractive, pink complexion. Women who smoke could save themselves the horrendous costs of beauty creams and of their cigarettes, *and* look far better by stopping smoking.

The rapid skin ageing induced by cigarette smoke is reflected in hormone levels, too. Women smokers have an earlier menopause than do non-smokers. Smoking businesswomen who plan to postpone their families until they are in their thirties may well lose out, permanently.

For older men and women, the main motivation to stop is health. The statistics regarding the survival of smokers beyond 60 are simply terrifying. A quarter of all men do not live to collect their pensions – smoking being the main cause of death in this group. If you are male and smoke and even this does not convince you to stop, at least think of your partner, who will probably be alone for the last 20 to 30 years of her life.

If you already have COPD, you have every reason to stop. If you continue, you will surely get worse, no matter how well your doctor and other carers treat you. How quickly you will deteriorate depends absolutely on how many cigarettes you smoke. Your *only* chance of feeling better, and being more physically active, is to stop. There could be no better motivation.

If you are caring for someone with COPD and you smoke, then *you* must stop, too. This is not only for your patient's sake – passive inhalation of someone else's smoke can greatly irritate damaged lungs – but for your own. You are no more immune to this disease, or all the other smoking-related diseases, than your patient.

How to stop

Once you are motivated to stop, you are well on your way to doing it, but how?

First make sure that your aim is to stop, not just to cut down, then be determined to do it, no matter what. In 1990, when I wrote a book on heart attacks, I was still advising people that they could choose between stopping suddenly and gradually. Now I am not sure that this is correct. In the intervening years, I have become convinced that the best way to stop is what I call the 'General de Gaulle method'.

General de Gaulle announced to the whole French nation, on television, that he had stopped smoking. After that, he never dared light up in case a member of the press caught him doing so and exposed him as a fraud or backslider! Most people could do something similar, in front of friends. In today's anti-smoking climate, such a move provokes sympathy and support, rather than sneers or sniggers.

I advise people to take all the cigarettes they possess – those in their pockets, handbags, home or anywhere else – scrunch them up, and throw them in the bin. Then to resolve never to buy any more, and always to say 'no', without thinking about it, to anyone who offers them one. As an extra, putting a non-smoking sticker on a window of the car and house can help.

People contemplating stopping suddenly always raise the question and the genuine fear of withdrawal symptoms. These can vary from agitation, irritation, nervousness and sleeplessness to nothing at all. I have found that people who have had to give up smoking for medical reasons, such as a heart attack, hardly ever have withdrawal symptoms, which strongly suggests that when they do occur they are psychological, rather than physical, in origin. If you have decided to stop because you want to improve the state of your lungs, I would wager long odds on that you will have no trouble. In any case, your desire to smoke will subside after a week or two as the feeling of wellbeing, caused by the dropping levels of carbon monoxide, nicotine and tar-linked chemicals in your blood and organs, takes over.

However, if you cannot stop completely in one go, try doing it gradually. Write your plan down and stick to it. Decide on a 'stop' day a few weeks ahead of time, preferably making it one during a long weekend off work or a holiday. Be aware of every cigarette smoked until that date and give each a value (in the range from one to ten) of its importance to you. You will then be able see how important smoking at that time of day is to you.

Keep your cigarettes in a drawer or on a shelf, not in a pocket or handbag, so that it is an extra effort to light one. Then, start your planned withdrawal by cutting out your 'best' cigarette of the day – the one that scored the highest. It may be the first one you have in the morning or the one that accompanies your morning coffee. Whichever one it is, *this* is the one you are likely to fail on. So, from the start, take special care not to succumb to it. Then, determine to delay your first cigarette of the day by one hour each day.

Carry chewing gum or low-calorie nibbles, such as pieces of carrot or celery, to chew when you feel the need for a cigarette. Get a friend to support and encourage you and monitor your progress every day. Use a graph to do this, if you wish.

If you find that you cannot stop, do not despair. Many people try several times before they finally succeed, and it gets easier with each effort. Your family doctor may help, with nicotine chewing gum and patches, or the drug Zyban, to stave off any withdrawal symptoms, but they are no substitute for a strong determination to succeed and the right motivation. If you use aids to stop smoking, understand that it still depends on *you*, not on the aid you have chosen or on anyone helping you. Chewing gum, acupuncture and hypnosis have no magical properties; they only support your own determination and cannot bolster a weak will.

As you stop, you must also understand that smoking has been a part of your life for years. You feel, rightly or wrongly, that it has helped you to relax or been a source of stimulus, so you must replace the feeling with another, just as satisfactory.

If you have COPD, finding such satisfaction is easy. You know that by stopping, you have just given yourself a good chance – your only chance – of a better life ahead. This in itself can be enough. However, you need to add to this a more positive attitude to life. It is a time to take more exercise, form new interests, take up new hobbies, even make new friends. These will all play their part in releasing tension and prevent you putting on too much weight. Your revived taste-buds (smoking weakens the senses of taste and smell) will give you so much more pleasure in eating that the thought of a smoke with or after a meal becomes repugnant.

From the time you reach the planned 'stop' day, the break must be complete. You will never buy or accept another cigarette. You will never risk 'just one', even at smoky parties where alcohol is flowing and your resistance is low. Be especially on your guard on such occasions. If you accept this one, you will be back where you started within weeks.

You owe the effort to stop smoking to your lungs and your future, and to the future of your partner and family. Even passive smoking hurts lungs, so everyone in contact with someone with COPD should stop, too. All the arguments that apply to people with this disease apply equally to everyone else, because no one knows when they will also be struck down by a smoking-related disease.

If you do stop, you will not be on your own. People in the UK are stopping smoking at a rate of around a million a year; only one adult in three or one in four now smokes. If you stop, you will be simply joining the sensible majority.

One vital aspect of becoming a non-smoker, if you have COPD, is to stop feeling guilty that you ever smoked. It is natural for someone who has a smoking-related disease to feel guilty about causing their own ill-health. As you almost certainly did not appreciate the consequences when you started, there is absolutely no point in feeling guilty now. Guilt wastes precious time, and just adds to the discomfort and inconvenience of the disease. Look on lung disease like the person who has developed heart disease from a faulty diet; no one blames themselves for eating a few extra cream cakes! Do not feel that you are to blame for your disease; just put your smoking years behind you and forget them.

Action on Smoking and Health (ASH)

In the first edition of this book, written in the mid-1990s, I spent several paragraphs saying how to avoid smoke in public places. Happily, in 2011, I've been able to delete them. In the UK now, smoking is banned from all public places, and we are all indebted to Action on Smoking and Health (ASH) for that fantastic change. ASH fought for many years for the right of non-smokers to breathe smoke-free air.

In October 1993, ASH launched its 'Breathing Space' campaign to create a more smoke-free environment in four areas of life: at work, in restaurants, cafés and pubs, in public places, such as banks and post offices, and in schools. The campaign was strongly supported by many health-related organizations, including the British Lung Foundation, and it was part of the Europe Against Cancer initiative, which was also launched in 1993.

ASH asked people all over the UK where their own smoke-free areas were and created a detailed library of where people can go and avoid other people's smoke. It was part of the process, still slow in the UK, but much more complete in Scandinavia and in North America, of enabling people to breathe uncontaminated air. The campaign was instrumental in the change in the law throughout the UK from 2007 onwards, which banned smoking in public places.

The benefits of stopping smoking

Finally, look at the following list of the benefits of stopping smoking and let it make your decision for you.

- Within 20 minutes of your last cigarette:
  - your blood pressure returns to normal
  - your pulse returns to normal
  - the temperature of your fingers and toes returns to normal.

- After eight hours:
  - carbon monoxide in the blood returns to normal levels
  - oxygen blood levels return to normal.

- After one day: the chances of you having a heart attack decrease.

- After two days:
  - your ability to smell and taste improves
  - your nerve endings start to work normally again.

- After three days:
  - your bronchi relax and open, widening the airways
  - your lungs expand, so that more air reaches the alveoli.

- After two weeks to three months:
  - your circulation improves
  - walking is easier
  - your lung functioning improves by a third.

- After one to nine months:
  - any cough, sinus congestion, fatigue or breathlessness decreases
  - the cilia regrow in your bronchi
  - mucus is cleared more effectively
  - your lungs are 'cleaner' and less prone to infection.

- After five years: lung cancer deaths fall from 137 to 72 per 100 000.

- After ten years:
  - lung cancer deaths fall to 12 per 100 000
  - rates of cancer of the mouth, gullet, bladder, kidney and pancreas decrease.

5

Treating COPD

Introduction

Now that you have put the problem of smoking behind you, we can start thinking seriously about treating all the forms of this disease.

The overriding aims of treatment are to reduce the excess mucus and cough of chronic bronchitis, to ease the breathlessness of emphysema, and to improve the patient's ability to exercise. Ways in which fitness can be improved by exercising are described in Chapter 3. This chapter covers other ways in which doctors and other professionals, such as physiotherapists, can help.

Surviving the winter

Many COPD sufferers dread the winter. They always feel worse in wintertime and they fear the episodes of infection, such as colds and flu, that, although a minor irritation to others, can be life-threatening for them. It is best to plan ahead.

The first rule is to keep warm. The best way to do this is to wear several thin layers of clothing through the day, not one thick layer. Clothes made from natural fibres (cotton, wool, silk) will generally keep you warmer than those made from synthetic ones. Keep your home warm, and take advice from your local gas or electricity showroom or real fire centre about getting the best from your heating system. At the same time, take advice on draught proofing your home.

Some heating systems make the air too dry for COPD sufferers. Personal humidifiers help, but a bowl of water near a radiator may be just as effective.

Eat at least one hot meal a day and take plenty of hot drinks in the meantime. Exercise matters, so if you cannot go outside, then exercise in the warmth at home. Walking up and downstairs – in your own time, and with rests when necessary – is good exercise, but even exercising your legs and arms while seated is better than nothing.

Keep extra medicines and inhalers in the home to use when bad weather keeps you housebound. Your doctor will advise you on their use. Keep another step ahead of the weather by listening to the weather forecasts before going out (see also Chapter 8 for sources of information). The Department of the Environment (DoE) has an Air Pollution Bulletin Service (see page 104 for the number), which forecasts pollution levels for each region and gives advice on what to do if the quality is poor (the BBC's Ceefax service has the same information in its weather section).

Other freephone helplines (for the numbers see page 104) include a Winter Fuel Line, the Warm Front Grants Helpline (for people who need help with insulating their homes) and a Benefit Enquiry Line (for people with any disability). Details of the benefits available to people with longstanding chest disease can be found in Chapter 9.

If you receive Income Support, a Council Tax rebate or Family Credit, you may be eligible for a grant from the Department of Energy towards insulating your home. Such a grant will help to cover the cost of insulating doors, windows, loft, pipes, and water tank. Simply contact Energy Action Grants Agency on the number given on page 104 for details of these grants.

If your income is low, you may be eligible for a grant from your local council. Such a grant could cover the cost of 'home renovation' which can include work from draught proofing to the installation of a central heating system. Councils differ in the kind of help they offer and the level of income and savings at which grants may be given.

Preventing infections – the importance of vaccines

The first priority for all COPD sufferers is to prevent lung infections, as repeated infections are a major cause of deterioration when a person already has bronchitis and emphysema. Two forms of vaccination can be helpful in this respect.

The first of these is the pneumococcal vaccine. This protects elderly people, in particular, against infection by pneumococcus, a bacterial strain that can cause severe bronchial infections and pneumonia in those over the age of 65. The standard recommendation in the UK is that all elderly people with COPD should be given a single dose of this vaccine.

Just as important is vaccination against influenza. Influenza viruses attack around a quarter of the population in any one winter. They are very difficult to control and monitor, as they pass among sea birds and pigs in the intervals between epidemics in humans, and they change their 'overcoats' as they do so. This means that the vaccines must be altered virtually every year, and that vaccinations must be repeated in susceptible people before the start of each winter.

To try to combat the right virus each season, most vaccines contain material made from three different strains of the virus – usually this means two types of 'A' virus, and one of 'B'. Vaccinating people with COPD against influenza, particularly older people, probably only reduces the chances of them catching influenza by about a third, but it almost certainly reduces the development of serious illness and complications, by 70 per cent. Also, in the UK, the Chief Medical Officer of Health, the most senior governmental medical officer, recommends to family doctors that they should vaccinate all people with chronic lung disease against influenza every year. Most years, the vaccines are ready by October or November in order to protect people against the expected outbreaks of the disease from January to March. Occasionally, as in the last quarter of 1993, the vaccines take longer to reach the pharmacies, and the virus arrives early. The result is a huge rise in severe chest illness among COPD sufferers and even some deaths.

Influenza itself causes few deaths, unless it is a strain that is particularly lethal. The 'Spanish' flu of the winter of 1918–19 is estimated to have killed more than 20 million people world-wide – 3 times as many people as were killed during the whole of the First World War! This pandemic, thankfully, was unique, and is not expected to be repeated, but severe epidemics of the 'A' virus type arrive every ten years or so, causing severe illness in millions of people and hundreds of thousands of deaths.

COPD makes you more susceptible than normal to the complications of influenza because your bronchi and alveoli are damaged, and their natural protection against infection is compromised. When the influenza virus hits the bronchi, the extra inflammation it causes makes the underlying tissues more susceptible to an added bacterial infection. These bacteria then multiply, to cause very severe illness. By preventing the influenza virus taking hold in the first place, such secondary bacterial infections are avoided.

So, if you have COPD, make sure you are on your doctor's flu vaccine list, and attend for your vaccination every October. It is well worth making the trip.

Treating the symptoms

Air pollution in your home

The pre-eminent everyday problem for those with chronic bronchitis is the constant production of excess mucus, and the cough that goes with it. Sufferers can help themselves by avoiding, as far as they can, the air pollution that plays a part in the irritation that precipitates the mucus production in the bronchi.

You can do little personally about the traffic pollution around you, except to avoid, if possible, being in the street at peak traffic hours. However, many people with bronchitis do not realize that the air in their homes can also be an irritant. The most obvious cause is tobacco smoke. The reasons for COPD patients not to smoke have all been given in the last chapter, but it is also important for guests to refrain from smoking in the house. A tactful explanation of why the house is a smoke-free zone should be enough for any visitor.

Animal dusts are another cause of irritation. Dog and cat hairs settle on carpets and furniture, and can cause long-term problems. The alternatives are very frequent and intensive vacuuming and cleaning – which can be exhausting for a COPD sufferer on their own – or not to have pets in the house. This can be very hard, especially if the pet is an old friend and a real source of comfort. At the very least, however, animals should be barred from the bedroom.

Moulds, mildew and bacteria caused by damp also irritate the airways of those suffering COPD. They may thrive in poorly maintained air conditioners or in poorly ventilated bathrooms and kitchens. The source of damp should be identified and corrected, and professional advice on how to effect efficient ventilation acted on.

Some people with this disease are sensitive to formaldehyde – a gas that can be released by some adhesives, carpets, upholstery fabrics and ply and particle board, used in building. It can cause headaches, dizziness, rashes and eye, nose and throat irritation. The air can be monitored for formaldehyde, and, if levels are high, the source can be removed, or covered with a coating. Improving ventilation also helps to overcome this problem.

Faultily installed gas and propane heaters and cookers can produce harmful amounts of nitrogen oxides and/or carbon monoxide – the same damaging gases that are produced by car exhausts. They, too, can irritate the lungs and cause headaches and nausea or more serious illness if they are not vented out properly. Any such appliance should be professionally installed and maintained, and have an outside vent. If you suspect that yours may be faulty, switch it off and contact your local gas board.

House dust mites are a powerful cause of wheezing in many people with COPD. They occur in every home, and are almost impossible to eradicate, unless you are prepared to live at an altitude of 1524 metres (5000 feet) or over as the mites do not survive above this altitude. However, the highest point in the UK is the summit of Ben Nevis, at 1341 metres (4400 feet)!

There are less drastic measures you can take, though, to lessen the problem. Mite populations can be reduced by frequently washing bed linen, quilts, pillows and blankets or using mattress and pillow covers that they cannot penetrate. Mites do not like low temperatures, so popping the pillows and quilts and any cuddly toys (often reservoirs of huge numbers of mites) into a chest freezer for 12 hours once a week may help.

Cleaning agents, pesticides, some personal care products and paints and solvents may also irritate the bronchi. If you need to use them, always follow the directions for their use very carefully, ensuring that there is good ventilation. Do not use aerosols.

You may have asbestos where you live – in lagging around pipes, water tanks and boilers, for example. If this is crumbling, it may be dangerous. Have it checked and make sure that it is only removed by specialists in asbestos removal (your local council will be able to advise you about this). Asbestos is also used in roofs, floors and insulation, but if it is in good condition and properly sealed, the risks of leaving it in place are tiny, compared with the real risk that would attend disturbing it. You should not drill, saw or sand down asbestos.

A final point about your home. If you have COPD, it is important to keep the air temperature at a reasonable level, say between 16 and 20°C (60 and 68°F), throughout the year. This is particularly important in the bedroom. Staying in a warm living room all day, then going to bed in a room containing cold air at night is asking for trouble because your chest will react badly to inhaling cold air. So be sure to keep every part of your home warm. If you cannot afford to do so, then either apply for a heating allowance from your local authority or move your bed into your living area for the duration of the cold weather. Cold air is just as much 'pollution' to COPD sufferers as dusty air.

Relieving coughs and reducing sputum

Different so-called cough medicines fill rows of pharmacy shelves. Unfortunately, they do not work, in the sense that they do not 'cure' coughs. Nor is it good to suppress a cough if you have COPD, unless it is a dry, irritating cough that keeps you awake, night after night. The cough is there to bring up sputum from the bronchi, so it is more important to help this process than it is to try to hinder it.

Cough medicines are classically split into 'expectorants', which help you clear phlegm, and 'suppressants', which shut down the cough reflex. There is no good evidence that expectorants actually work better than breathing in steam or drinking plenty of water (2–3 litres/3½–5¼ pints a day). On the other hand, cough suppressants *do* stop a cough, but this leaves potentially infected phlegm inside the chest – not a good idea for anyone, let alone COPD sufferers. A dose of a cough suppressant, such as linctus codeine, last thing at night, to prevent your sleep being disturbed by constant coughing, is probably the only valid medical reason for taking a cough medicine.

If you start to produce too much phlegm (say more than a third of a cupful a day) then you may be developing problems other than uncomplicated COPD, and you should see your doctor. If they are ruled out, you may be prescribed drugs known to reduce sputum volume, such as atropine or steroids. 'Beta-mimetic' bronchodilator drugs, such as salbutamol, or lung stimulants, such as theophylline, may be prescribed to help open the airways and clear them of mucus.

Treating bronchial infections

Bacteria thrive in the bronchial mucus and from time to time, in every person with COPD, they overpower the body's immune defences against them. The result is a chest infection or, more accurately, an infection in the bronchi. The medical phraseology for this is an 'acute exacerbation of chronic bronchitis', and this is what is usually written on certificates of absence from work due to sickness.

You know that you have an acute infection when you feel hot and sweaty, weak and tired, cannot stop coughing, find it difficult to breathe, even at rest, and your phlegm has become thick and yellow or green. You may have a pain in the ribs or throat as a result of coughing, but as your lungs do not contain pain-sensing nerves, you may not feel any pain in the chest.

Bouts of acute bronchitis often follow colds. These are virus infections of the nose and throat, and are shaken off in a few days, without complications, by most people. If you have COPD however, colds often leave the bronchial tree more susceptible than usual to 'secondary' invasion by bacteria. So, the lesson for sufferers of this disease is to avoid people in the first three days of a cold (when they are spreading the virus by coughing and sneezing), and people with colds should postpone visits to anyone with a 'bad chest' until they are back to normal health.

If you have COPD, as soon as you know you are developing acute bronchitis, contact your doctor, who will prescribe an appropriate antibacterial drug. Many doctors prefer to give prescriptions in advance, so that their patients with this disease can start the treatment as soon as they feel unwell. This saves valuable time, and can greatly reduce the severity of, and shorten, the acute infection.

Antibacterial drugs are of two main types: antibiotics, derived from cultures of moulds that naturally prey on bacteria, and synthetic antibacterials, derived from other chemicals.

The first synthetics, the sulphonamides, originated from chemical (aniline) dyes. However, today's first-line drugs, used to combat acute bronchitis, include penicillin-like antibiotics, such as ampicillin and amoxycillin, and antibiotics unrelated to penicillin, such as tetracycline and erythromycin. Trimethoprim is a first choice synthetic antibacterial.

If, within 48 hours, these drugs have not made you feel substantially better, the sputum has not returned virtually to normal and you are still distressed by breathlessness and coughing, then you will be given second-line, more powerful, drugs. Among these drugs are 'cephalosporins', (such as cefaclor, cefuroxime, and cephalexin) 'aminoglycosides' (amikacin, gentamicin) and 'quinolones' (ciprofloxacin). Table 2 in Chapter 10 gives the trade names of these drugs.

The vast majority of bouts of acute bronchitis respond very well to a course of antibiotics, and most of the rest quickly respond to a second prescription. The small number that do not do so need specialist attention in hospital, where not only will more antibiotics be given, but the patient will be given oxygen to breathe, and specialist drugs to support the heart and remove excess fluid from the lungs (for more details of this kind of treatment, see pages 74–5).

Physiotherapy and postural drainage

Physiotherapy is sometimes recommended as a means of helping people with an acute bronchial infection to 'get the phlegm up', but the experts disagree on how effective it is. Trials have failed to show much benefit, and it is felt that percussing (gently slapping) the chest and using vibration techniques can actually worsen the obstruction of air flow in some patients with COPD. However, I have to say that I am strongly in favour of physiotherapy. I have seen physiotherapists have considerable success in coaxing thick and plentiful mucus out of patients with acute infections that would not otherwise come out. Many people swear by (and sometimes at) their physiotherapist, and I would not like to argue with them!

One group of these patients – those with bronchiectasis – *definitely* benefit from physiotherapy. Pummelling the chest wall helps them to get rid of their excess mucus. In particular, they benefit from what is termed 'postural drainage'. In many cases of bronchiectasis, the damage is confined to one area of the lungs, usually near the base of each lung, just above the diaphragm. It is difficult to cough phlegm upwards from here, so the trick is to position yourself in such a way that you can cough *downwards*, gaining the help of gravity, instead of fighting against it. Thus, if the base of your right lung is affected, lie on your left side, with your hips and legs on your bed or sofa, and your upper body bending over the side towards the floor, with your head near the floor and your mouth over a bowl on the floor. Then, cough downwards in this position, several times. You will find that the mucus from the base of the lung flows much more freely than if you tried to cough up. If your left lung is affected, lie on your right side and repeat this process.

Many people with COPD, find postural drainage useful even when they do not have bronchiectasis. However, if you do this do it with caution and when advised to do so by a physiotherapist, especially if you have heart problems.

Drugs that improve your air flow

Once the diagnosis of COPD has been made, your doctor will want to know how well your lungs can respond to drugs to reverse any asthma-like reaction.

In asthma, the muscles in the bronchi are constricted, narrowing the airway, causing difficulty in breathing, especially in breathing out. The standard treatment for asthma today is to prescribe a combination of drugs to reduce the inflammation that occurs in the bronchi due to allergy and to relax the constricted muscles.

The drugs are taken via inhalers, so that they reach the site of the problem, deep in the lungs, and only minute amounts of them get into the general circulation or to other organs. This is important as full doses of both types of drug given by mouth could produce serious side effects. For example, the steroids that simply reduce the inflammation when taken by means of an inhaler could otherwise make you put on unwanted weight, weaken bones and make you more susceptible to infections, among other problems. The 'bronchodilator' drugs to relax the bronchi, such as salbutamol, which just relax the bronchi when inhaled, could otherwise cause the heart to race – not desirable if the heart is already trying to cope with your lung disease. Happily, the dose delivered by an inhaler of either type of drug is too small to cause these effects. It must be remembered that COPD is *not* asthma, so inhalers are not going to be the complete answer to any sufferer's problems; they will not completely abolish coughing or breathlessness. However, in virtually everyone with the disease there is some asthma-like activity in the bronchi. They are inflamed, and the bronchial tree, though not in severe spasm, as in an asthma attack, is often 'tight' and could open up if the muscles were able to relax more. So, doctors often prescribe bronchodilator inhalers for patients who have COPD to try to improve the flow of air through the bronchi, marginal though the improvement might be.

Bronchodilators

The most commonly prescribed bronchodilators are salbutamol and terbutaline. The standard inhaler doses of these two drugs (usually two puffs three or four times a day) do not affect the heart, but users should understand that if they are exceeded, they may develop palpitations or feel their heart racing. If they do, they should consult their doctor. Other possible side effects from taking too high a dose include shakiness (tremor), cramps and agitation.

Longer-acting bronchodilators, such as salmeterol and formoterol, have been devised that only need to be given twice a day. This is useful for people who wake in the night breathless as the effect of these drugs lasts all night.

'Anticholinergics'   These are also bronchodilators, but they work better on the larger airways than on the middle-sized to smaller ones, which is ideal as it is these larger airways that are the main cause of trouble in COPD. They are slower to act than salbutamol or terbutaline (taking from half an hour to an hour to work), but the effect lasts for six to eight hours. One advantage they offer is that they can dry up the mucus better than other bronchodilators, and the two types can be used together to better effect with a lower dose of each.

Ipratropium and oxitropium used to be the two most prescribed anticholinergics. The inhaler preparations of these have few side effects, but when given in high doses, usually in nebulizers (see Chapter 6), they can affect the ability of the bladder to empty in susceptible people, blocking off the flow of urine. Also, anticholinergics have a bitter taste, which some people find impossible to tolerate. (See 'A new anticholinergic', page 69).

'Methylxanthines' In the nineteenth century, one of the foundations of the treatment of COPD and asthma was black coffee because strong coffee opens wheezy airways. This is because it contains the 'methylxanthine' theophylline. Theophylline and other methylxanthines do help air flow and stimulate the activity of the lungs in asthma, but they are less useful in the treatment of COPD.

Drugs containing theophylline are swallowed, not inhaled. They all have the drawback that the dose has to be very carefully monitored and adjusted by the doctor as side effects are common at doses only a little higher than the dose needed to produce a beneficial effect. If you feel sick, actually vomit or cannot sleep because the drug makes you feel too wide awake, then your dose is too high. Serious reactions to theophylline include abnormal heart rhythms and epileptic fits, so if you are prescribed a drug containing theophylline, be very careful to follow the instructions regarding dosage to the letter.

There are now 'sustained release' forms of theophylline, the effects of which last for 12 hours. They are to be taken last thing at night to reduce coughing and wheezing in the small hours of the morning. To reduce side effects, especially in older people, the treatment is started with a low dose, which is slowly increased over two or three weeks.

Using an inhaler

Although using an inhaler is the best way to deliver drugs to the lungs, as many as half of all inhaler users do not operate them correctly. Most of the powder or liquid intended for the lungs, in fact, is swallowed, which defeats their object.

Inhaled treatment can be administered in four main ways: by metered dose, spacers and nebulizers. All aim to deliver around 10 per cent of each dose deep into the lungs. Not doing this properly, which lowers the percentage of the drug getting there even further, will obviously make the treatment much less efficient.

Metered dose inhalers With this type of inhaler, you must co-ordinate your intake of breath with the release of the dose from the inhaler in the following way:

1 Remove the cap from the inhaler and shake.
2 Hold the inhaler upright between your thumb and forefinger.
3 Tilt your head back slightly.
4 Breathe out.
5 Put the mouthpiece of the inhaler in your mouth and close your lips around it.
6 Begin to take a deep, slow breath in, through your mouth, and activate the inhaler by pressing down on the canister while continuing to take the deep inward breath.
7 Hold your breath for 10–15 seconds.
8 Breathe out slowly, then wait one to two minutes before taking the second puff.

Some inhalers are activated by the act of inhalation. This was meant to get round co-ordination problems, but patients can still find them difficult.

Spacers These are tubes or cones attached to metered dose inhalers and are designed to help people who cannot co-ordinate their breathing with the activation of the inhaler. The dose is released into the spacer chamber and you then inhale it from the mouthpiece. Spacers should deliver around 20 per cent of a dose into the lungs. Older patients who have COPD and children who have asthma find them useful.

Nebulizers In nebulizers, pumps are used to drive air containing a moisturized cloud of drug into a face mask around the nose and mouth. They deliver around 15 per cent of a dose of the drug to the lungs. Many people now use nebulizers at home, with considerable benefit. However, they must be supervised closely and there needs to be fast access to service and technical facilities if things go wrong or materials run out.

In the UK, nebulizers are offered free on loan from local District Health Authorities when hospital consultants consider they are necessary for a particular patient. However, in many districts, all the nebulizers are constantly out on loan or broken or only available for short periods. The British Lung Foundation successfully campaigned for nebulizers to be available on National Health Service prescription, but many charities, like Lions Clubs and Hospital Leagues of Friends, still buy them for hospitals to lend to patients at home.

When you start using a nebulizer, you may find the pump motor a little noisy, so you may find it difficult to fall asleep for the first few nights. One of my patients dealt with this by pretending to herself that it was a railway engine. She had never found it difficult to sleep on a night train and, when she closed her eyes, she imagined she was doing just that! Others have drowned the noise by playing their favourite music. Whatever method you use, if you do find it difficult to begin with, persevere as the brain has a way of denying a persistent noise after a time and you will soon settle into a normal bedtime routine again.

Steroid treatment

Steroids (corticosteroids), such as cortisone or prednisolone, are very useful in treating asthma, in which they suppress the allergic reaction of inflammation in the bronchi. They are less useful in treating COPD however, as infection and structural damage to the bronchi are the main problems. Nevertheless, a few patients who are 'chronic bronchitics' do also have some asthma. Most doctors therefore feel that patients who have COPD should at least have a trial period using an inhaled steroid, such as beclomethasone or budesonide. The steroid trial can only be started when the person is in a stable condition, with no infection. The results of PF measurements and six-minute walk tests are recorded in a patient diary, and repeated every day for two weeks. The improvement in the results of the tests at the end of this time determines whether or not they should continue to receive this treatment. If the PF levels do improve (an increase of at least 25 per cent would be expected) then the steroid inhaler treatment can continue, but in addition to the other treatment. Some doctors, however, prefer to do the initial trial with high doses of a steroid (prednisolone) by mouth for a few days (too short a time to give rise to serious side effects), then, when the result is positive, to switch to the inhaled beclomethasone or budesonide afterwards.

However the trial is performed, in long-term inhaled steroid treatment, the doses for COPD patients are usually higher (around eight puffs per day) than those needed for asthma (two to four puffs per day). At doses of over eight puffs per day, the usual side effects associated with steroids can arise, so anyone prescribed inhaled steroids for their COPD must not exceed the recommended dose, even by as little as a couple of puffs. Regular use of high doses of a steroid can cause problems in the throat, such as thrush infections, so if your throat starts to dry up or to ache when you are taking it, see your doctor.

Treating disabling breathlessness

Some people who have had COPD for years find that they are breathless all the time, even seated at home, doing nothing, and despite having had all the treatment mentioned so far. They may benefit from low doses of opiate drugs, which slow down and deepen breathing, and more importantly, perhaps, reduce your own perception of your breathing. They slow down the whole body's metabolism, reducing the need for oxygen.

Drugs of this type include dihydrocodeine and methadone. If you need this kind of medication, you will need to go to hospital to start your treatment, under specialist supervision, which will commence after blood tests have shown that the oxygen levels in your blood are lower than normal. People who have to take these drugs for long periods may find that they feel sick, and they can cause constipation and sleepiness, so the dose must be very carefully chosen to give the best possible relief from the feeling of breathlessness, while minimizing the risk of side effects.

Coming to terms with depression

It is entirely understandable that around half of all people with chronic lung disease are depressed. Dependency on others, loss of self-esteem, preoccupation with their breathing and fear of the future all play their part.

One way to combat this is to aim for the sky – to be as energetic as possible, and to aim to return to as many normal activities as possible. Your physiotherapist will help in this by giving you a training programme that suits you, as an individual, and by encouraging you. Your improvement may be simply the result of using your muscles more effectively, rather than an actual improvement in your lungs, but this does not matter because you will feel better, regardless of the cause of this feeling.

It is important to exercise every day until you reach a state of breathlessness. It will not do your lungs any harm and it is encouraging to find that you will have to exercise more, week by week, in order to become breathless.

If, despite such efforts, you cannot shake off your depression, your doctor may prescribe an antidepressant drug that will not make you drowsy or weaken your ability to breathe, such as desipramine or fluvoxamine.

The need for oxygen – respiratory failure and the heart

Sometimes COPD becomes so severe that you need more oxygen than you can get from the air you breathe. This state may arise during an acute exacerbation of bronchitis and emphysema or it may result from a more gradual problem and your heart has simply begun to show the strain. Whatever the cause, you will need oxygen therapy. The next chapter describes this state of respiratory failure and what can be done if it occurs.

A new anticholinergic — 2001 update

In 2001 a third anticholinergic, tiotropium (Spiriva), was made available to doctors. This has the big advantage over the others that the benefits of one dose (in terms of improving lung function tests — see pages 29–31) last a full 24 hours after each dose. In the detailed and large trials of tiotropium there were no side effects at any dose. These results strongly suggest that tiotropium may well replace ipratropium and oxitropium within a few years.

6

When you need oxygen

Introduction

In the later stages of COPD (sadly, mainly reached by people who could not stop smoking) the lungs are too damaged to keep oxygen levels in the blood high enough for comfort. The heart tries to compensate for the lungs' failure by enlarging, in an effort to drive more blood through the lungs. The effort is in vain as the problem is not the lack of blood, but the failure of the lungs to maintain enough air flow to the alveoli.

Symptoms of respiratory failure

Doctors used to divide people at this stage of COPD, rather unkindly, into 'pink puffers' and 'blue bloaters'. The pink puffers mainly have emphysema. They look breathless, even when resting, although they may not feel as if they are breathless. They tend to breathe through both the nose and mouth, and to use their shoulder and neck muscles with every breath. Whether or not they feel that they are breathless at rest, they become quickly distressed by their breathlessness on the slightest exertion. They tend to be underweight, with sunken cheeks and hollow eyes. They only become blue ('cyanosed') and their legs only begin to swell with fluid very late in the course of their illness.

The blue bloaters, in the main, have had chronic bronchitis. They go blue very easily, especially in the lips and cheeks. They are usually overweight and tend to have swollen feet and ankles, but they neither look nor feel as breathless as the pink puffers. They can usually manage a little exercise before they 'run out of puff', but, when they do, their cheeks and lips can become quite blue, even violet.

Some people with chronic lung disease also develop finger 'clubbing', which is when the ends of the fingers expand and the nails bulge outwards. This is a sign of chronic sepsis in the lung or of a longstanding lack of oxygen to the tissues. It is generally found in those who have bronchiectasis and other lung and heart problems, but also in people with chronic bronchitis, indicating that they have complications that need to be investigated.

The pink puffers and blue bloaters are stereotypes of the two extremes of the same disorder. Most COPD sufferers in the late stages of the disease seen by general practitioners like myself exhibit features of both types of failure, and we are always on the lookout for signs of this. Symptoms of impending lung failure include swollen ankles, rapidly worsening breathlessness, a steep reduction in the amount of exercise that can be taken, a bounding pulse, and headaches and periods of confusion.

Blood tests show an increase in the numbers of red cells – yet another mechanism the body uses to try to compensate for the lack of oxygen. Particularly important, though, is the measurement of oxygen and carbon dioxide levels present in blood taken from an artery. Falling oxygen levels (hypoxaemia) coincide with rising carbon dioxide levels (hypercapnia). The lack of oxygen causes confusion, temporary loss of intellect and sleep disturbances. The high carbon dioxide levels cause headaches, shaking and, eventually, severe sleepiness in the daytime.

The treatments

If the first attack of respiratory failure coincides with an acute bronchial infection, then antibiotics are given to combat the germs, diuretics are given to get rid of any excess fluid and reduce the strain on the heart, and bronchodilators, such as salbutamol, are given by nebulizer or even directly by injecting it into a vein to open the congested airways. Sometimes high doses of steroids are given, also by injection into a vein.

Oxygen treatment

The main need in such cases is oxygen. It is given either by means of nose prongs or a mask, starting at low flow levels and building up gradually, according to the levels of oxygen in the blood. Too much oxygen must not be given too soon as the sudden change may make the breathing control centre in the brain shut down altogether, which would mean that spontaneous breathing would stop.

Such 'controlled oxygen therapy' has enabled most patients developing acute respiratory failure during a bout of acute bronchitis to survive and recover without the need to place them on ventilators – machines that force air into and out of the lungs. Ventilators are usually reserved for patients who had, before their acute illness, reasonably good lungs, but which are now overwhelmed by, say, pneumonia.

Once the patient has recovered from a first attack of respiratory failure (and the vast majority of patients who have COPD do so), it is time to review the treatment and the desirability of giving oxygen permanently.

The modern use of oxygen in treating this disease stems from two hospital trials that took place in the UK and the USA between 1975 and 1980. The Medical Research Council's trial in the UK allocated people who had had at least one attack of respiratory failure to either treatment with controlled oxygen therapy or without it. All the other treatments – antibiotics, diuretics and bronchodilators – were the same for all the patients. The oxygen was given by nasal prongs for at least 15 hours every day. After three years, there were 50 per cent more survivors in the group receiving oxygen therapy than in the group not given oxygen.

The US study compared groups of patients given oxygen for 12 hours, mainly at night, with those given oxygen round the clock (in reality around 19 hours a day). The trial was stopped after 18 months because survival among the patients receiving oxygen treatment for 12 hours a day was much lower than that in the group receiving oxygen treatment for the longer period.

A more recent study of 72 patients in Sheffield has confirmed that oxygen given for at least 15 hours per day gives up to five years of extra life to patients who have COPD.

In addition to improving survival, these studies all showed that oxygen therapy improved patients' psychological state and intellect, extended their ability to exercise, lessened breathlessness and improved the quality of sleep.

Providing an oxygen service

These international studies have proven beyond doubt that oxygen must be provided for people with advanced COPD. Most countries have already set up home oxygen services. In the UK, oxygen concentrators are the preferred device, but are very expensive.

An oxygen concentrator is a machine that converts the air around it into a stream of at least 90 per cent oxygen. The oxygen is delivered into the nostrils by two small tubes at a rate of about 2 litres per minute. This is usually enough to correct the low blood oxygen level of most patients who have COPD who are experiencing chronic lung failure. Oxygen should be given for at least 15 hours in every 24, including the whole night.

The machine is placed conveniently in a porch, hall or spare bedroom, and stiff plastic tubes carry the oxygen to the living and bedrooms, where there are terminals to which the cannulae (tubes for the nose) can be attached. The doctor or nurse visits at least once a month to discuss the treatment, encourage the patient and to read the time clock, checking that the 15-hour a day treatment is being maintained.

Like nebulizers, oxygen concentrator pumps are noisy, and people can take time to get used to them. One emphysema sufferer has his own particular way of coping with this aspect.

> It reminds me of a plane engine and let's face it, in a plane that is a welcome sound because if you couldn't hear it you'd be in trouble. I lie in bed and imagine I'm flying above the earth to an exotic paradise, to a holiday in the sun or just a fantasy world before I drop off to sleep. At bedtime I almost look forward to taking off on my dream flight. Well, it works for me, but then I'm a little mad. In my business, you have to be mad or you'd go crazy!

In the UK patients can only be selected for home oxygen treatment if they have low oxygen levels in their arterial blood – breathlessness without such hypoxaemia is not an acceptable criterion. Before being accepted, patients must also be non-smokers. Amazingly, many people are still smokers when they reach the stage of lung failure! Obviously, smoking in a house containing an oxygen concentrator is a considerable fire hazard, but, apart from this consideration, the carbon monoxide in the blood of smokers completely nullifies the effect of oxygen, making the treatment useless. Once you start oxygen treatment, it needs to be continued for the rest of your life.

Some people prefer masks to the cannulae, but they are less suitable for long-term use because they must be removed for eating, drinking, talking and coughing up phlegm and, anyway, many mask types are simply not suitable for use with oxygen concentrators. It is best to get used to cannulae if possible.

Portable oxygen is available in lightweight gas cylinders that last around 40 minutes. They give housebound patients the chance to venture out, though not very far afield. Portable liquid oxygen gas units mean you can travel further, but they are far more expensive than the gas cylinders and, as fewer than half of all patients who have COPD and are receiving regular oxygen treatment ever go out of doors, they have not been widely accepted.

'Short' oxygen treatment

Oxygen cylinders are still bought from pharmacists by COPD sufferers who believe that an *occasional* deep breath of oxygen will relieve their breathlessness. Sadly, there is no good evidence that it does and, in most patients, the perceived benefit is no better than that after a breath from a cylinder filled with normal air.

For some people their daytime blood oxygen level is normal, but it dips steeply while they are asleep. This may be a sign of poorer health to come. They may be prescribed oxygen through the night, but, although it may improve the blood test result, it does not seem to improve the quality of their sleep.

Assisted ventilation

A small number of people are unable to breathe independently after an acute attack of lung failure, so their breathing may need to be assisted for the rest of their lives. We now have home 'intermittent positive pressure ventilation' (IPPV) machines for them. These pass air through a tracheotomy tube (which is inserted through a hole made by a surgeon in the throat just underneath the larynx) into the lungs at pressures equivalent to the pressure we exert on the lungs when we breathe normally. People who have their breathing assisted in this way require skilled nursing and constant attention, which few families can provide for long.

Lung transplants

The ultimate treatment for chronic lung failure is, of course, a lung transplant. Although for some patients a single lung transplant is feasible, the usual operation for lung failure is a heart and lung transplant, in which the whole chest cavity is virtually emptied and the organs replaced by those from a donor. Obviously it is a major operation with many attendant risks and only undertaken when there is no alternative. When it is successful, as it was, for example, for the neurosurgeon and MP from Glasgow Dr Sam Galbraith, it can give years of useful extra life.

The drawback for patients who need this operation is that donor organs are in very short supply. The main source used to be road traffic accidents, but the legislation that made the wearing of seat belts compulsory has (thankfully!) greatly reduced the numbers of potential donors. This has meant that transplants have been restricted to younger people with the most serious diseases, such as teenagers with cystic fibrosis, and younger adults with progressive massive fibrosis of the lung (a condition in which both the lungs are massively affected by fibrous scarring), which was the case for Dr Galbraith.

COPD sufferers are unlikely to be placed on a transplant list unless they have reached the final stages of the disease before their forties, which is very unlikely. Of course, if you are still smoking, having a transplant is unthinkable as the risks of surgery are much higher, and the new lungs will quickly be affected by the same disease that caused you to need the transplant in the first place.

A final thought on oxygen

I cannot let this chapter end on such a sad note. If you are now dependent on oxygen, there are still ways in which you can enjoy life. Probably the most heartening story I have heard is that of Eric Coombe.

> Mr Coombe is 74. He has been paralysed for 23 years, and now has heart trouble and breathing difficulties. He has to take his oxygen wherever he goes, which is quite a way! Eric has an electric Mobibuggy, which is a cross between a wheelchair and a small car, that is fitted with a 1360-litre oxygen cylinder. He can visit friends and relatives, using the oxygen as necessary, even when travelling on pavements or roads.
>
> He repairs clocks and watches for the blind, cooks Sunday lunch for his family, and videos wildlife on his buggy rides. The buggy battery can last 16 kilometres (10 miles) on one charge, and he regularly drives 8 kilometres (5 miles) a day.

Further, a letter from 'K. W.' of Cambridgeshire shows the sort of spirit that really makes my heart lift. She wrote to *Breathing Space*'s readers:

> May I implore you not to turn it [the Breathe Easy network] into a self-pity society?
>
> I was once told by a specialist that nothing more could be done and I must live with it. Fortunately my young doctor didn't agree with him and I am now on oxygen therapy and still alive and kicking. Despite being 79 years old and having to be pushed around in a wheelchair, I find life quite enjoyable. Please, all you 'gaspers', keep your sense of humour. You will find people more helpful if you do.
>
> My motto is *dum spiro spero* – while I breathe I hope. May I suggest the Breathe Easy network adopt it too?

There could not be a better attitude to COPD and I recommend it wholeheartedly.

7

Your 'home team'

Who they are and what they can do for you

Whether or not you are eligible for benefits, a 'home team' is ready to help you if you have chronic lung disease. It includes the general practice team of your doctor and receptionist, health visitor, nurse, social worker, occupational therapist and physiotherapist. The reorganization in the National Health Service has meant that more decisions are being taken at general practice level than before and this may be an advantage to COPD sufferers, as the power to make decisions is devolving to the people who know the patients best – their practice's professionals.

The team's first priority is to make life as normal as possible for you. The team's expertise means that it can give advice on your ability to work and how to change working practices to suit your physical capabilities as well as organize nursing and home aids to make routine chores easier and less energy-sapping.

Sadly, I have to agree that in the past – even the recent past – doctors tended to accept that there was little to be done for the patient with COPD. It was common to certify a patient unfit to work for repeated three-month periods, prescribe the usual combination of drugs, give some advice about smoking, and leave the patient to their own fate.

Happily, in most general practices this is no longer the case. Nurses in practices run chest clinics for asthmatics and patients who have COPD, checking their PF scores and diaries, taking time to talk about particular problems, and working out the best ways to solve them.

Organizing nebulizers and oxygen concentrators is only a small part of the team's job. Other examples are the provision of a home help or visits from Meals on Wheels for people whose breathlessness makes it difficult for them to cook or do housework. Telephone rentals may be paid where a person lives alone who is at risk of sudden illness – a very real threat for someone in the later stages of COPD.

Nursing aids can be provided, such as incontinence pads, pants and sheets, and other devices for women whose lives are being made less than happy by urine leakage when they cough. The occupational therapist can arrange for handrails to be put in on stairs, or for baths to be converted into walk-in showers. Financial help may be arranged for damp houses to be treated or, sometimes, in the case of council house tenants, for patients to move to another house or flat. Alternatively, swaps between upstairs and downstairs flats may be organized. Oxygen-carrying transport, where necessary, can be ordered for hospital visits. Voluntary workers can be contacted to sit with patients while a partner goes out shopping or to take the sufferer shopping or just for a pleasant trip out.

Sex

Regular contact between medical professionals and patients who have COPD builds up confidence and you can get to know each other very well. This is the time when more delicate issues, like a couple's sex life, may be raised.

Many couples give up on their sex lives too early. The partners of patients hold back because they feel that the exertion may be harmful, even precipitate lung or heart failure. The patient may feel that they are unattractive and that their partner will not be interested. These feelings can be well wide of the mark.

The practice team will be happy to give advice on ways in which you can make love that will not put excessive strain on the partner with the disease and will make it a satisfying experience for both of you. Finding ways in which you can become a loving, even passionate, couple again can be a great boost to both patient and carer.

Taking care of the carer

The practice team recognizes, of course, that it is just as important to look after the carer's needs as it is to look after those of the patient. Months of caring for someone, no matter how much you love them, who is constantly coughing, producing copious, frankly disgusting, phlegm, and who is distressingly breathless on the slightest exertion, saps the patience of even the most saintly. To this add all the noise and paraphernalia of the nebulizer and oxygen concentrator, and the labour involved in the simple acts of going to the toilet, washing, dressing and undressing, and the carer's life can seem like a nightmare from which there is no escape.

The COPD sufferer can do much to help them. Most important is to be positive and cheerful, even when you do not feel like it. The second is to do as much as you can to keep up appearances, so, if you are male, then be clean-shaven, smell good and dress well. If you are female, put a little make-up on, keep your hair in good condition, dress attractively and put on some perfume. Be as tidy as you can be, and help where you can. Always remember that exercise is better than rest, so if there is any household chore you can do, do it, even though it makes you a bit breathless. All these things will make you feel better and your carer will be happier. Even though the effort tires you out, it is worth it, and in the long run, it will make you fitter and better able to fend off the challenge of future chest infections.

If you are a carer, your practice team will understand any feelings you have of fear, disgust, resentment and depression. You are not alone in this and no one will blame you for them. Once they are brought into the open and you know that they are entirely normal reactions to the strain, not something to feel guilty about, you can begin to deal with them in a constructive way. You can do this in various ways, from arranging a regular day off or a holiday or, if the illness is very severe, a 'respite care' fortnight in a local hospital specializing in such cases.

8

People, organizations and going places

The British Lung Foundation

I have mentioned the British Lung Foundation and its Breathe Easy network and I have no hesitation in putting it at the top of my list of organizations who can help people who have COPD and their families.

The British Lung Foundation exists to promote research into, and help people with, lung diseases. Its founders were distinguished academic chest physicians, but its list of Vice-Presidents includes people from all walks of life, among them mountaineer Chris Bonington and diplomat Lord Tugendhat. Others included Nobel Prizewinner Sir Douglas Black and world-renowned medical statistician Sir Richard Doll.

Doctors and researchers at more than 30 top British hospitals and universities are currently benefiting from grants from the Foundation. Many of them are studying the prevention, diagnosis and treatment of bronchitis, emphysema, and bronchiectasis. To give some examples of this work:

- In Nottingham, researchers found that diet may help to cause or prevent COPD (emphysema may be linked with diets low in vitamins C and E or lacking in copper and selenium).
- In London's National Heart and Lung Institute, the Foundation's funds are helping to determine how a lack of oxygen affects various body tissues.
- At the Hammersmith Hospital, the Foundation supports research into the nature of the inflammation in chronic lung disease.
- In Cardiff, researchers are unravelling why some people are particularly at risk of developing bronchitis and emphysema.

The British Lung Foundation, through the Breathe Easy network, is a powerful lobby for better treatment of lung patients by the government. For example, campaigns have included one to make nebulizers available on the National Health Service, one concerning improving disability benefits, and one regarding combating air pollution. This last campaign covers concerns about the levels of ozone in summer in cities – a considerable cause of acute lung inflammation – and other such concerns. Professor Stephen Holgate, a vice-president of the Foundation, did much to make the problem of city air pollution known and chaired the Department of Health's pollution advisory group. Under his guidance, the Foundation funded major research into the link between pollution and lung disease.

The British Lung Foundation has regional offices and Breathe Easy self-help groups, so if you have COPD or care for someone who has it, you will find that help is available locally (see page 103 for an address and phone numbers).

One of the best of the Foundation's projects is their free newspaper *Breathing Space*. Published four times a year, it is also available online through the British Lung Foundation Breathe Easy website. Many of the case histories in this book have been drawn from its lively accounts. The *Breathing Space* newsletter and Breathe Easy network aim to help people with COPD to communicate with each other and to dispel their feelings of isolation. The newsletter gives up-to-date information on the latest treatments and services, and campaigns for improved facilities for, and public understanding of, the problems faced by people with breathing difficulties. Since it was started in 1991 by Trevor Clay, former Secretary General of the Royal College of Nursing, it has attracted more than 12 thousand regular readers. This sounds like a lot of people but this is only a tiny proportion of the million or more people in the UK who have COPD. So, if you had not heard of the British Lung Foundation or Breathe Easy before, join up now. You will learn a lot about your illness and about how you can do much to help yourself and others with similar problems. Sadly Trevor died in April 1994. Living as he did with emphysema, he launched Breathe Easy to provide a positive public face for lung disease and to give it a voice that could not be ignored by government, Members of Parliament, health professionals and the general public. His legacy lives on.

One disturbing fact discovered by the Breathe Easy team is that many people with this disease are a little disenchanted with their doctors, who should be the main helpers in the lives of those with a chronic illness. Time and again the *Breathing Space* postbag has contained letters containing comments like; 'My doctor has no time for me' or 'He says nothing can be done'.

The Foundation responded quickly to this by drawing up an action plan on how to get the best from your doctor. The plan gives details of how to prepare the subjects you wish to discuss at your consultation beforehand, advises taking a relative with you for support, and when and how to involve the practice nurse. It also advises that it is a good idea to take a list of the medicines you are taking with you. The Foundation suggests that as most doctors work in group practices, there may be one doctor who has a particular interest in chest disease; so it is worth asking about this and then seeing him or her. There may also be a 'chest' nurse, who could advise on everyday problems. Patients who have COPD may wish to ask about lung function tests, nebulizer and oxygen treatment and flu vaccines. If these questions are written down beforehand, it helps the flow of the consultation with the doctor and ensures that you cover everything you want to know about. Breathe Easy will send a copy of their action plan to any interested person (for the address, see page 103).

Breathe Easy has also helped to set up scores of local support and self-help groups for people with COPD and their families. For people wary that such groups may meet just to wallow in mutual self-pity, it would appear that this is very far from the truth! Contact Breathe Easy at the British Lung Foundation's London address on page 103 for more information.

Chest Heart and Stroke Scotland

Scotland is fortunate in that it has two very strong charities working for people with chronic chest disease in this part of the country. One is the British Lung Foundation, mentioned above, which has interests and responsibilities throughout the UK. The other is Chest Heart and Stroke Scotland. Like the British Lung Foundation, Chest Heart and Stroke Scotland spends much of its income on supporting medical research in hospitals and universities but concentrates its efforts just in Scotland. It also distributes welfare grants to elderly people with chest disease, a service arising from its origins in the National Society for the Prevention of Tuberculosis. It also prints leaflets advising people on chest diseases, including COPD, and sponsors self-help 'chest groups'. If you want to find out more about this organization you will find their address on page 103.

Getting out and about and going on holiday

There are enlightened organizations that are happy to cater for people with COPD, among them the National Trust and the Royal Society for the Protection of Birds.

Under the National Trust's Access For All Scheme, over 200 properties have facilities for people with special needs. A guide to them is available from National Trust shops or from the address given on page 104.

More than 20 of the Royal Society for the Protection of Birds' British reserves are suitable for disabled visitors. They prefer to receive advance warning of your visit (contact details given on page 105).

Among a number of holiday companies specializing in helping people with lung conditions are those given on pages 104 and 105.

Holiday information services

Eurolung Assistance has a directory of oxygen equipment companies in different countries, of clinics and hospitals able to assist in emergencies, and services offered by airlines to people needing oxygen. Breathe Easy will provide this information (see page 103 for their address).

These are only a few of the organizations that have formed to help the disabled enjoy a break away from their own four walls. Breathe Easy will certainly have details of many more, so if you wish to spread your wings, contact them.

Looking after yourself

To make the best of your planned break, stick to the following guidelines.

- Discuss your plans with your doctor, who will guide you on what you can do and what, perhaps, you should avoid. They may be able to give you advance prescriptions, to avoid the catastrophe of running out of your treatment while you are away.
- If you use a nebulizer or oxygen, let your hotel and airline know well in advance, so that it can be organized to cater for your needs.
- If you need a wheelchair, the local branch of the Red Cross will provide one. Your hotel will wish to know beforehand, so that you have a chair-friendly room and toilet.
- Take out the appropriate insurance. Some policies do not cover people with pre-existing disease. Cover your special equipment against loss or damage, too, and insure beforehand against having to cancel or shorten your holiday.
- If you are staying in the EC, apply for a European Health Insurance Card (EHIC) by calling 0845 606 2030 or going to the website <www.ehic.org.uk>. This entitles you to medical care in most EC countries.
- Most airlines say that they will provide oxygen, but be careful they know beforehand that you will need to use it for at least 15 hours in every 24. Some charter companies do not accept people who need oxygen to this extent on their flights, and even some scheduled flight operators will balk at the mention that someone needs to use it for more than 2 hours during a flight. Contact their medical department before booking the flight.
- Consider seeking financial help. Your Social Services department (Social Work department in Scotland) may be able to give assistance, and some charities help defray holiday expenses for the disabled.

- Finally, have courage and go for it! Most travel companies and hoteliers are happy if they know your problems and needs in advance.

9

Claim what you are entitled to

Introduction

The Government provides some help for people with disabilities, but this is mainly designed for people with more obvious handicaps than 'chronic chests', such as blindness, paralysis or mental impairment. It is often difficult – much too difficult, really – for COPD sufferers to be successful in their claims.

Benefits available to people with COPD

There are three major allowances for the disabled: the Disability Living Allowance, the Attendance Allowance and the Disability Working Allowance.

Disability Living Allowance

This is a tax-free benefit for people who need help with personal care, such as washing, dressing and cooking, or with moving about or both. It is for people who became disabled before they were 65, and is paid even when they live alone and do not have help. It can be claimed by anyone under 65 or before you reach 66.

You must usually have needed help for three months, and be expecting to need help for at least another six months. Very seriously ill people may qualify under the section headed 'Special rules'. All you need to back your claim is for your doctor, nurse, occupational therapist or physiotherapist to fill in the appropriate section on your claim form. You do not need a medical examination.

The Allowance consists of a weekly amount to be used to cover care needs and a weekly amount to help with mobility. Both the care and mobility benefits can be set at different rates and paid to the same person. The benefit does not depend on your savings or your income and should not affect any other benefits you may be claiming.

Attendance Allowance

This allowance is also tax free and is designed to help people over 65 who need assistance with personal care, in exactly the same way as does the Disability Living Allowance, even if you are not actually receiving help. To qualify for it, you must normally have been ill for at least six months, but, like younger people given the Disability Living Allowance, if you are seriously ill you may receive it sooner under the special rules.

There are two rates at which Attendance Allowance can be paid – a smaller amount if you need care in the daytime *or* at night, or a larger amount if help is needed both day *and* night.

Disability Working Allowance

This is a tax-free benefit for people who can still work, but whose illness or disability limits the amount they can earn. You can claim it if you have been put at a disadvantage in finding a job, because of your illness or disability, if you are looking for work for the first time or you are already working at least 16 hours a week. You must also already be receiving a DWP benefit for illness or a disability.

The Allowance is given for 26 weeks, after which you must renew your claim. You do not normally need a medical examination to claim it but it does depend on your other income and savings. It may reduce the amount of any housing benefit you may be receiving, but not the Disability Living Allowance. Also you cannot receive Family Credit and Disability Working Allowance at the same time. (To find out more about all these benefits, see page 104 for the phone number of the Benefit Enquiry Line.)

The future

Sadly, at the time of writing, it is difficult for people with COPD to qualify for the higher levels of benefits or for mobility allowance, as most are mobile for short periods and, for example, have enough breath to make a meal. Yet, sufferers have to rely far more than the rest of the population on friends or taxis to travel very short distances, such as to the shops or to the doctor's surgery, which makes life very expensive if you want to maintain your independence.

The failure of authorities and the staff of many public services to recognize the limited mobility of the people who have this disease is a recurring concern of readers of *Breathing Space.* Many write in who have received no mobility allowance, many have even had difficulty obtaining the orange wheelchair badge signifying a disabled driver, and many find the staff in public places cater well for people in wheelchairs, or who are blind or deaf, but have little understanding of, or apparent sympathy for, people who are standing up but plainly out of breath.

The British Lung Foundation and Breathe Easy are trying to change this image. Their campaigns for an improvement in attitudes and for much better provision of equipment such as nebulizers and oxygen concentrators for people with chronic lung disease may make a difference. Let us hope so, because the tenth of the British population who have COPD deserves a much better deal.

10

Prescriptions for COPD

The different types of medicines prescribed for COPD were described in Chapter 5. The most commonly prescribed current drugs are listed in more detail in Table 2 overleaf, with their prescription (generic) and proprietary (trade) names. They are in alphabetical order, not in order of preference.

Table 2 Drugs commonly prescribed for COPD

Type of drug	Generic name	Trade name
Antibacterial	amikacin	Amikin
	amoxycillin	Amoxil
	ampicillin	Penbritin, Amfipen
	cefaclor	Distaclor
	cefuroxime	Zinnat
	cephalexin	Ceporex, Keflex
	ciprofloxacin	Ciproxin
	doxycycline	Vibramycin, Nordox
	erythromycin	Erythrocin, Erymax
	gentamicin	Gidomycin, Genticin
	oxytetracycline	Imperacin, Terramycin
	tetracycline	Achromycin, Tetrabid
	trimethoprim	Monotrim
	(+ sulpha)	Bactrim, Septrin
Bronchodilator	bambuterol	Bambec
	fenoterol	Berotec, Duovent
	formoterol	Atimos, Foradil, Oxis
	salbutamol	Ventolin,
		Ventodisks,
	salmeterol	Volmax
		Serevent
	terbutaline	Bricanyl
Xanthine (lung stimulant)	aminophylline	Phyllocontin
	theophylline	Choledyl, Nuelin, Slo-Phyllin
Anticholinergic (to reduce mucus)	ipratropium	Atrovent, Duovent
	tiotropium	Spiriva
Steroid (against inflammation)	beclomethasone	Becloforte, Becotide,
		Becodisks, Ventide
	budesonide	Pulmicort
	fluticasone	Flixotide
Cough medicines Suppressants*	codeine	Benylin Dry Cough
	codeine	Calpol, Phensedyl
	dextromethorphan	Actifed Co
Expectorants*	pseudoephedrine	Actifed expectorant, Sudafed

*There are many other cough suppressants and expectorants, most containing mixtures of drugs.

11

The perspective from 2010: how we manage COPD today

In July 2010, *Drugs and Therapeutics Bulletin* (*DTB*), an independent journal produced for British doctors by the *British Medical Journal* group, published an editorial review of all the evidence on preventing exacerbations in COPD. The *DTB* is sent to all doctors practising in the UK each month. It is very highly respected, and deservedly so, for its unbiased analysis of the choices that doctors have in making decisions for our patients.

For GPs, its conclusions are invaluable, as they cover all aspects of treatments for common ailments – no mean feat, as we are bombarded almost every day with the launch of new products and new claims for old ones. For a working GP, it is often difficult to keep up with them and, when we do, it is difficult for us to judge which claims are justified and which are not. So the *DTB* is a must read for practising doctors.

The editorial in the July 2010 issue of *DTB* comprehensively covered the modern management of COPD, starting with the Global Initiative for Chronic Obstructive Lung Disease (GOLD) established in 2009.

GOLD defines COPD as a 'preventable and treatable disease characterised by airflow limitation that is not fully reversible [in which it differs from asthma], and that results in debility over time'.

To translate that into layman's language: COPD makes it difficult for you to breathe deeply and easily, and the difficulty gets greater as it progresses. We can't reverse the process, but we can slow it down, and even, perhaps, stop further deterioration.

We understand now that the deterioration isn't a gradual, constant, continuing, insidious process. It is driven by 'exacerbations' – periods when your lungs are infected and inflamed. With each episode the lungs are damaged a little, so that the more exacerbations you experience the worse your baseline lung function becomes. If we can avoid this stepwise fall in your ability to breathe, we can keep you as well as possible.

Dealing with exacerbations professionally and successfully is therefore the most important service we GPs can offer you. We need, as far as possible, to prevent them, and if there is a breakthrough exacerbation, to treat it effectively and successfully.

How do you recognize an exacerbation? You won't have any doubt. Your breathing is much worse, you are producing a lot more spit than normal and it is often yellow or green, and thick. You are hot and sweaty. I don't need to describe the way you feel: if you have COPD, you will know from bitter experience of past bouts of what we used to call 'acute bronchitis' what it is like.

The first priority for you, therefore, is to prevent any more exacerbations. Is there evidence that any of the drugs you take (they are discussed in Chapter 5) do so? This is where I am so grateful to the *DTB*. In its 2010 review of COPD management, all the well-controlled trials of the treatments we offer came under scrutiny, some with surprising results. I've summarized the conclusions here, so that you can judge for yourself how well you are managing your own COPD. It is essential that you are part of the decision-making process of the medical and nursing team that is looking after you, and that you know why we are prescribing your particular medicines.

Chapter 5 dealt with the drugs that you are likely to be prescribed by your family doctor. This chapter reviews the up-to-date evidence for why we prescribe them. As with all long-term illnesses, it's helpful if you know as much as you can about why you are being asked to take them. If you know the reasons for taking your medicines, you are more likely to do so with confidence.

I'll start with the two commonest: the bronchodilators and the steroids. The trial results strongly suggest that the bronchodilator of choice for prevention of exacerbations of COPD is the long-acting drug salmeterol. Given twice daily in a 50-microgram dose, it reduces the numbers of exacerbations per year by around 15 per cent: put another way, if four people are treated for a year, it will prevent one exacerbation. That may not sound much, but it is a significant improvement for many COPD sufferers.

This was a similar effect to that of inhaled steroids (see Chapter 5), in which the average fall in exacerbation numbers was around 18 per cent. However, giving inhaled steroids alone, long term, in COPD has serious adverse effects. Among them are thrush in the throat and a constantly hoarse voice. They are even linked to a slightly higher risk of pneumonia. The UK Medicines Regulatory Agency has warned us not to prescribe inhaled steroids on their own.

Combining salmeterol with an inhaled steroid doesn't seem to help better than just using the salmeterol alone. The difference in results between giving the two together and giving the broncho-dilator alone was too small to be of real benefit. Nor was there any advantage in taking the combination of bronchodilator and steroid over taking the drug tiotropium (see Chapter 5) alone. When all three drugs – salbutamol, a steroid and tiotropium – were taken together, they were no more effective in preventing exacerbations than when just one of them was taken.

Tiotropium is an anticholinergic drug (see Chapter 5). Anticholinergic prescribing has changed since the first edition of this book. These drugs have one advantage over the other bronchodilators: they dry up the mucus inside the chest more effectively, so your chest seems to be 'clearer' than without them. However, they act on other secretory systems, too, so that they can cause bladder problems, give a dry mouth and eyes, and even in a few people, constipation. These side effects are thankfully rare, and as a GP of many years' standing, I must admit that most patients report that they have had absolutely no bother with them. Ten years ago, the standard anticholinergic was ipratropium (Atrovent): a newer drug then, with longer action, was oxitropium. Today, oxitropium has gone, and its place on medical schedules has been taken by tiotropium (Spiriva), also with a longer action than ipra-tropium. Many GPs still prescribe ipratropium, and although the latest clinical trials suggest that the longer-acting drug should be more effective, I can see their point in not replacing the tried-and-trusted drug, especially when their patients find it useful, with the newer one.

There are other theoretical choices for preventing exacerbations. Trials of 'mucolytic' drugs – drugs designed to thin the mucus produced by lungs affected by COPD – have shown that they lower numbers of exacerbations by about one every two years per patient, but perhaps only in patients who are not using a steroid inhaler. Whether this is worthwhile is questionable: the official advice to doctors (from the British National Formulary) is that that they should be stopped if the patient sees no benefit after taking them for four weeks. Current mucolytics include carbocisteine, erdosteine (Erdotin) and mecysteine (Visclair).

Another approach to preventing exacerbations is to take a daily antibiotic. Some doctors reserve this for patients with advanced COPD who are constantly becoming infected. It is doubtful that this really makes a difference, and it isn't officially recommended. However, once the exacerbation has started, and you know that you are having one of your 'ill turns', then an antibiotic is essential. Many GPs, myself included, will prescribe a course of antibiotics in advance for patients with regular exacerbations, to start as soon as their next exacerbation begins.

As winter approaches, our COPD patients are advised to have their annual influenza vaccine: we often write out the 'wait-and-see' antibiotic prescription described in the previous paragraph at the same time. Although influenza is a virus infection, and therefore not susceptible to ordinary antibiotics, the damage it does to the lung leaves it open to a superinfection with the usual bacterial suspects – and a full-scale exacerbation, often with pneumonia, will ensue.

Regular flu vaccinations are therefore essential for all people with COPD, and there is good evidence that they really do protect against exacerbations. The *DTB* report quotes, from the 2009 Cochrane Database Systematic Review (the bible of clinical trial assessments), a study by Dr P. Poole and colleagues which concluded that flu vaccinations reduced exacerbations of COPD by around a third. Interestingly, vaccine against the pneumococcus (the once-only vaccine against pneumonia) had no effect on exacerbation rates.

Managing your own COPD

All the advice on medicines for COPD given in the last few pages will only help you as long as you also understand how much you can do yourself to reduce your risks and improve your lung function. The most important message for you is that, even when your lungs are working at less than half their potential capacity, you can do a lot to improve them, over and above taking your prescribed medicines.

The Cochrane system of trial reviews reported in 2008 that 'pulmonary rehabilitation' programmes for COPD patients are safe and effective in lowering their number of future admissions to hospital. Rehabilitation introduces you to a gradual increase in exercise, teaches you about your illness, improves your psychological approach to it and changes your behaviour to eliminate, as far as possible, your risks. Naturally, if you smoke, stopping is the first priority in rehabilitation.

Rehabilitation systems are not set in stone: they are adapted to each patient's needs, and even, dare I say, to the personalities of the staff conducting them. They are organized and led by nurses specially trained in COPD and its problems. I am privileged to work as a regular locum doctor in several practices, and find them to be exceptionally effective. The patients are so much better informed about their illness, and do so much better, because they understand why they are being asked to follow the team's advice. By recognizing when they need to start their antibiotic, or perhaps a steroid inhaler, they can keep most of their exacerbations at bay, and consequently cut down their hospital admissions and the length of time for which they are ill.

I've found that little things can matter a lot. After the first edition of this book was published, I was asked to speak to a meeting of the West Midlands branch of Breathe Easy. After my talk the lively audience discussed at length the best pieces of advice they had been given over the years. The one I remember still, fifteen years later, I use for all my COPD patients. It is simply to buy a packet of toy balloons, and every morning to blow up three or four of them (see page 33). You will love it. It is often difficult to muster up enough 'puff' to begin with, but once you start to achieve a full-blown balloon you will not look back. Over the months your lung function should gradually improve, and you will be less breathless. Many of my patients have surprised themselves by how much further they can walk after starting on the balloon exercise.

Your nursing lung rehabilitation team will know of many more ways to help you move onwards: take the advantage of following their advice. It is an addition, not an alternative, to your medical treatment, and you will enjoy the regular contact with staff who really care about improving your health in a kindly and sympathetic way.

NICE 2010

I can't finish this chapter without referring to NICE, the National Institute for Health and Clinical Excellence in England, Wales and Northern Ireland. In 2010 NICE upgraded its recommendations to doctors for managing COPD. Here they are:

- Everyone with COPD who still smokes should be encouraged to stop and offered help to do so at every opportunity. The age does not matter: even in old age, stopping smoking will lead to some improvement.
- If you are constantly breathless and have exacerbations on the usual inhaled bronchodilators, but still have more than half the expected lung capacity, you should be given a long acting beta-agonist bronchodilator such as salmeterol or a long-acting anticholinergic such as tiotropium. If your lung capacity has fallen below the halfway mark you should be given the choice of a combined inhaler of a bronchodilator and steroid or of a bronchodilator and an anticholinergic.
- If you are still breathless despite the combination of a bronchodilator and a steroid, an anticholinergic should be added, regardless of your lung capacity.
- Everyone with COPD should be offered pulmonary rehabilitation.

I am fortunate that I work in an area (South West Scotland) where we do offer pulmonary rehabilitation: it is spreading widely. If it is not available in your area, please take up the subject with your local practice. It is a vital addition to your continuing good health.

Glossary

acute A sudden, short, usually severe illness. In bronchitis, it usually signifies an episode of infection, that needs antibiotic (and perhaps oxygen) treatment.

airways The whole system that enables us to breathe, from the nose to the alveoli, through the throat (pharynx), past the larynx, through the trachea (windpipe) to the bronchi and bronchioles.

alpha-1 antitrypsin A substance normally present in the tissues, an inherited lack of which causes emphysema in a small number of people.

alveolus (plural, alveoli) The air sacs deep in the lung where oxygen from the air enters the blood circulation and carbon dioxide passes from circulation into the air. The many 'leaf' ends of the 'branches' that make up the bronchial 'tree' (we have more than 300 million alveoli). They are damaged in emphysema, usually by smoking. A few people inherit alveolar disease – *see* alpha-1 antitrypsin.

antibacterial A group of drugs that fight infection. They are made from chemicals rather than from living sources, such as moulds. Sulphonamides and quinolones, such as the active drugs in Septrin and Ciproxin, are antibacterials.

antibiotic A group of drugs that fight infection. Purified from moulds, they include penicillin, tetracycline or cephalosporins.

anticholinergic A type of drug designed to dry up mucus and help open large airways. Examples are atropine, ipratropium and tiotropium.

antitussive A cough suppressant medicine. Most antitussives contain codeine or a similar drug to 'shut down' the centre in the brain that is responsible for initiating coughing in response to an irritant in the airways. Antitussives are of doubtful value in chronic lung disease.

asbestosis A lung disease caused by breathing in asbestos fibres. It varies in severity from mild COPD to fibrosis and cancer of the lung. Asbestos is a mined mineral used in fireproofing.

aspergillosis A fungus the spores of which (often from mouldy hay) can cause chronic lung disease if inhaled.

asthma An illness in which the bronchi are oversensitive to impurities and respond by becoming inflamed and narrowing. Both reactions can be reversed by steroid and bronchodilator inhalers.

betamimetic A type of bronchodilator drug, such as salbutamol or terbutaline.

bronchi The main branches of the respiratory 'tree'. They carry air to the alveoli, and are the site of infection and excess mucus production in bronchitis.

bronchiectasis A disease in which some segments of the bronchi are wider than normal and produce too much mucus. This leaves the lung open to infections and COPD.

bronchioles The smallest bronchi, nearest the alveoli. Their delicate lining membrane can be badly damaged by smoking. Can be infected in children, in bronchiolitis, caused mainly by a bacterium (Haemophilus influenzae). Early bronchiolitis may be the forerunner of later chronic bronchitis.

bronchodilators Drugs that open up the bronchi. Used mainly in the treatment of asthma, they can help some people with COPD.

byssinosis A chronic severe COPD-like lung disease caused by breathing in air contaminated by cotton dust that is also known as 'Cotton worker's lung'.

carbon dioxide A waste gas formed as a result of the body's energy processes. It is expelled through the alveoli as they take in oxygen. It builds up in the blood if the lungs fail; *see* hypercapnia.

chronic Medical term for a long-term illness: the converse of acute.

COPD Chronic obstructive pulmonary disease, previously called chronic obstructive airways disease. Usually a combination of chronic bronchitis and emphysema that leads to coughing and breathlessness. Almost always associated with smoking.

cilia Microscopic hairs that line the bronchi and move in unison, like waves, to cause mucus to flow up and out of the lungs. They are greatly damaged by smoking and repeated lung infections. Some people with COPD have inherited cilia that do not work efficiently – *see* Kartagener's syndrome.

cor pulmonale Heart strain complicating chronic lung disease. Symptoms include breathlessness, ankle swelling, tiredness, and lack of energy.

diuretic Drug that acts to remove excess fluid from the body. Used to ease cor pulmonale.

dust disease Lung disease caused by dusts, which can be industrial, due to air pollution, or biological, from grains, moulds, bacteria, animal dander, feathers or excreta. Found in miners, stonemasons, farmers, bird fanciers, and people from other occupations.

dyspnoea Medical term for breathlessness.

emphysema Disorder in which the alveoli are distorted, so that the oxygen and carbon dioxide transported across their walls are reduced. The main sign of this is breathlessness (dyspnoea).

exacerbation A sudden worsening of bronchitis and emphysema symptoms, usually due to a chest infection.

expectorants 'Cough medicines' that aim to loosen phlegm and make it easier to cough it out. There are doubts as to whether or not they work.

fibrosis A process of scarring throughout the lungs that reduces their normal ability to recoil when breathing out. It leaves people very breathless after the slightest exercise. Sometimes associated with dust diseases, but the cause may never be found. Cystic fibrosis is an inherited disease in which the mucus in the bronchi is far thicker than usual, there is great difficulty in coughing it out, and the lungs are especially prone to infection.

hypercapnia A condition in which there is too much carbon dioxide in the blood. It occurs when the lungs are failing.

hypoxaemia The condition of there being too little oxygen in the blood – another sign of lung failure.

influenza A virus infection that attacks the bronchial tree. Outbreaks occur in most winters and COPD sufferers are particularly susceptible to serious acute illness after a flu attack.

influenza vaccine A vaccine made from current influenza viruses that aims to protect against the next outbreak.

inhaler Device designed to deliver drugs directly into the airways.

Kartagener's syndrome A form of inherited lung disease in which the organs are on the opposite side to normal and the cilia do not work properly.

McLeod's syndrome A form of inherited emphysema in which there are ciliary problems, but the organs are on the correct side.

methylxanthine A drug that stimulates the lungs and opens airways. Examples are theophylline and choline theophyllinate (Choledyl).

nebulizer A system that delivers drugs to the lungs in a 'cloud' of vapour.

oxygen Gas in the air essential to every body process. It enters the circulation through the alveoli. When the lungs begin to fail, oxygen levels in the blood fall (hypoxaemia).

oxygen concentrator An electrical device that produces a flow of 90 per cent oxygen from normal air (which is 23 per cent oxygen). The method of choice for oxygen delivery to patients who have COPD in the UK.

pneumoconiosis 'Miner's lung'. Any disease in which mineral dust has damaged the lungs, but it is usually applied to coalminers.

psittacosis 'Bird fancier's lung'. A dust disease caught from inhaling the feather dust or excreta of birds.

pulmonary rehabilitation Treatment aimed at improving lung function using long-term exercises and lifestyle advice and changes, alongside prescription medicines.

respiratory Adjective pertaining to breathing. The 'respiratory tract' is the medical term for the airways and 'respiratory failure' is lung failure, in which there is hypoxaemia, hypercapnia and breathlessness at rest.

ventilator Machine used to keep the lungs breathing when they have failed. Usually electrically driven, they apply pressure intermittenly inside the lung.

xanthine The group name for methylxanthine drugs.

Useful addresses

Action on Smoking and Health (ASH)
First Floor
144–145 Shoreditch High Street
London E1 6JE
Tel.: 020 7739 5902
Website: www.ash.org.uk

British Heart Foundation
Greater London House
180 Hampstead Road
London NW1 7AW
Tel.: 020 7554 0000
Heart HelpLine: 0300 330 3311 (9 a.m. to 6 p.m., Monday to Friday)
Support Care Team: 0844 847 2787
Website: www.bhf.org.uk

British Lung Foundation and Breathe Easy
73–75 Goswell Road
London EC1V 7ER
Tel.: 020 7688 5555
Helpline: 08458 505020 (10 a.m. to 6 p.m., Monday to Friday)
Website: www.lunguk.org

Alternatively, phone one of their regional offices:
Midlands: 0116 249 5780
North: 0191 263 0276
North West: 0151 224 7778
Scotland and Northern Ireland: 0141 248 0050
South West: 0117 300 4080
Wales: 01792 455764

Chest Heart and Stroke Scotland
65 North Castle Street
Edinburgh EH2 3LT
Tel.: 0131 225 6963
Advice line: 0845 077 6000 (9.30 a.m. to 4 p.m., Monday to Friday)
Website: www.chss.org.uk

Alternatively, there are offices in Glasgow and Inverness:
Glasgow: 103 Clarkston Road, Glasgow G44 3BL; tel.: 0141 633 1666
Inverness: 5 Mealmarket Close, Inverness IV1 1HT; tel.: 01463 713 433

Department of the Environment's Air Pollution Bulletin Service
Tel. (freephone): 0800 556677

Department for Work and Pensions (DWP)
Winter Fuel Line: 0845 9151515 (8.30 a.m. to 4.30 p.m., Monday to Friday)
Benefit Enquiry Line: 0800 882200 (8.30 a.m. to 6.30 p.m., Monday to Friday; 9 a.m. to 1 p.m., Saturdays)
Website: www.direct.gov.uk
www.dwp.gov.uk
For all advice on care and benefits for people who are disabled or chronically ill and their carers. Includes advice on employment and job support.

Energy Action Grants Agency (EAGA)
EAGA House
Archbold Terrace
Jesmond
Newcastle-upon-Tyne NE2 1DB
Tel.: 0191 247 3800
Warm Front Grants Helpline: 0800 316 6011
Website: www.eaga.com

Help the Handicapped Holiday Fund (3H Fund)
B2
Speldhurst Business Park
Langton Road
Speldhurst
Tunbridge Wells
Kent TN3 0AQ
Tel.: 01892 860207
Website: www.3hfund.org.uk
Organizes holidays where volunteers and nurses travel with disabled people in groups of up to 30 within the UK and abroad.

National Trust
PO Box 39
Warrington WA5 7WD
Tel.: 0844 800 1895
Website: www.nationaltrust.org.uk
The National Trust provides access to its properties and facilities for disabled visitors.

Royal Society for the Protection of Birds
The Lodge
Potton Road
Sandy
Bedfordshire SG19 2DL
Tel.: 01767 680551
Website: www.rspb.org.uk

Society of Teachers of the Alexander Technique (STAT)
First Floor, Linton House
39–51 Highgate Road
London NW5 1RS
Tel.: 020 7482 5135
Website: www.stat.org.uk
STAT (as it likes to be called) has a brilliant website. Phone the office and speak to either Ilia or Lesley, or email <office@stat.org.uk>.

Tourism for All
c/o Vitalise
Shap Road Industrial Estate
Shap Road
Kendal
Cumbria LA9 6NZ
Tel.: 0845 124 9971
Website: www.tourismforall.org.uk
Helps people with chronic illnesses and disabilities find appropriate and supported holidays.

Index